MEDICAL INTELLIGENCE UNIT

Molecular Mechanisms of Fanconi Anemia

Shamim I. Ahmad, B.Sc., M.Sc., Ph.D.
School of Biomedical and Natural Sciences
Nottingham Trent University
Nottingham, England, U.K.

Sandra H. Kirk, B.Sc. (Hons.), Ph.D.
School of Biomedical and Natural Sciences
Nottingham Trent University
Nottingham, England, U.K.

Landes Bioscience / Eurekah.com
Georgetown, Texas
U.S.A.

Springer Science+Business Media
New York, New York
U.S.A.

MOLECULAR MECHANISMS OF FANCONI ANEMIA

Medical Intelligence Unit

Landes Bioscience / Eurekah.com
Springer Science+Business Media, Inc.

ISBN: 0-387-31972-7   Printed on acid-free paper.

Copyright ©2006 Eurekah.com and Springer Science+Business Media, Inc.

All rights reserved. This work may not be translated or copied in whole or in part without the written permission of the publisher, except for brief excerpts in connection with reviews or scholarly analysis. Use in connection with any form of information storage and retrieval, electronic adaptation, computer software, or by similar or dissimilar methodology now known or hereafter developed is forbidden.
The use in the publication of trade names, trademarks, service marks and similar terms even if they are not identified as such, is not to be taken as an expression of opinion as to whether or not they are subject to proprietary rights.
While the authors, editors and publisher believe that drug selection and dosage and the specifications and usage of equipment and devices, as set forth in this book, are in accord with current recommendations and practice at the time of publication, they make no warranty, expressed or implied, with respect to material described in this book. In view of the ongoing research, equipment development, changes in governmental regulations and the rapid accumulation of information relating to the biomedical sciences, the reader is urged to carefully review and evaluate the information provided herein.

Springer Science+Business Media, Inc., 233 Spring Street, New York, New York 10013, U.S.A.
http://www.springer.com

Please address all inquiries to the Publishers:
Landes Bioscience / Eurekah.com, 810 South Church Street, Georgetown, Texas 78626, U.S.A.
Phone: 512/ 863 7762; FAX: 512/ 863 0081
http://www.eurekah.com
http://www.landesbioscience.com

Printed in the United States of America.

9 8 7 6 5 4 3 2 1

Library of Congress Cataloging-in-Publication Data

Molecular mechanisms of Fanconi anemia / [edited by] Shamim I. Ahmad, Sandra H. Kirk.
    p. ; cm. -- (Molecular biology intelligence unit)
  Includes bibliographical references and index.
  ISBN 0-387-31972-7 (alk. paper)
  1. Fanconi's anemia--Genetic aspects. 2. Fanconi's anemia--Molecular aspects. I. Ahmad, Shamim I. II. Kirk, Sandra H. III. Title. IV. Series: Molecular biology intelligence unit (Unnumbered)
  [DNLM: 1. Fanconi Anemia--genetics. WH 175 M718 2006]
RC641.7.F36M65 2006
616.1'52071--dc22
                            2005037313

CONTENTS

Preface vii

1. **Clinical Features of Fanconi Anaemia** 1
   A. Malcolm R. Taylor
   Genetics of Fanconi Anaemia 2
   Clinical Features of Fanconi Anaemia 3
   Fanconi Anaemia and Nijmegen Breakage Syndrome 5
   Confirmation of the Diagnosis in FA Patients 6
   Relationship of Complementation Group to Clinical Features ... 7
   Evidence for Modifying Mutations 10

2. **The Genetic Basis of Fanconi Anemia** 13
   Grover C. Bagby, Jr.
   Genetic Heterogeneity 13
   The *FANC* Genes 14
   FA Protein Complexes 21

3. **The *FANCA* Gene and Its Products** 28
   Laura S. Haneline
   FANCA Gene 28
   FANCA Protein 29
   FANCA Function 30
   Acquired AML and FANCA Defects 32

4. **The *FANCC* Gene and Its Products** 36
   Susan M. Gordon and Manuel Buchwald
   Cloning and Characteristics of the *FANCC* Gene 36
   Mammalian Homologs of FANCC 37
   FANCC Gene Mutations 39
   Expression of the FANCC Gene Products 40
   FANCC Protein Expression and Stability 41
   FANCC Subcellular Localization 41
   FANCC in the Cellular Response to ICL Inducers 42
   Apoptosis 43
   FANCC Loss of Function 43
   FANCC and Cytokine Signalling 45
   FANCC and Oxidative Stress 47

5. **The *FANC B, E, F* and *G* Genes and Their Products** 54
   Filippo Rosselli
   FANCB 55
   FANCG 56
   FANCF 57
   FANCE 57

6. **FANCD1/BRCA2 and FANCD2** 61
   Gary M. Kupfer
      The FA-D Complementation Group 61

7. **The *FANC* Genome Surveillance Complex** 67
   Takayuki Yamashita
      Historical Overview 67
      Structure of the FA Core Complex 69
      Functions of the FA Core Complex 70
      Perspectives 71

8. **Other Proteins and Their Interactions with FA Gene Products** 74
   Tetsuya Otsuki and Johnson M. Liu
      FANCC-Binding Proteins 74
      FANCA-Binding Proteins 75
      FA Protein Complex and Human α Spectrin II 78

9. **Fanconi Anaemia and Oxidative Stress:
   Cellular and Clinical Phenotypes** 82
   Giovanni Pagano and Shamim I. Ahmad

10. **Therapy for Fanconi Anemia** 92
    Madeleine Carreau
       Androgens 92
       Hematopoietic Growth Factors 92
       BM Transplants 93
       Gene Therapy 96
       Prospects for Therapy 98

11. **Mutational Analyses of Fanconi Anemia Genes
    in Japanese Patients** 103
    Akira Tachibana
       Patients, Cell Culture and Mutation Analysis 103
       Sequence Variations in the *FANCA* Gene 104
       Sequence Variations in the *FANCG* Gene 108
       Mutations of the *FANCC* Gene 111
       Mutations of Other FA Genes 111
       Characteristics and Genetic Basis of Japanese FA Patients 111

   Index 115

EDITORS

Shamim I. Ahmad
School of Biomedical and Natural Sciences
Nottingham Trent University
Nottingham, England, U.K.
Email: shamim.ahmad@ntu.ac.uk
Preface, Chapter 9

Sandra H. Kirk
School of Biomedical and Natural Sciences
Nottingham Trent University
Nottingham, England, U.K.
Email: sandra.kirk@ntu.ac.uk
Preface

CONTRIBUTORS

Grover C. Bagby, Jr.
OHSU Cancer Institute
Departments of Medicine
　and Molecular and Medical Genetics
Oregon Health and Science University
Portland, Oregon, U.S.A.
Email: grover@ohsu.edu
Chapter 2

Manuel Buchwald
Department of Molecular
　and Medical Genetics
University of Toronto
Toronto, Ontario, Canada
Chapter 4

Madeleine Carreau
Department Pédiatrie
Université Laval
Unité de Recherche en Génétique
　Humaine et Moléculaire
CHUQ, Pavillon St-Francois d'Assise
Québec, Québec, Canada
Email: madeleine.carreau@crsfa.ulaval.ca
Chapter 10

Susan M. Gordon
Program in Genetics
　and Genomic Biology
Research Institute
Hospital for Sick Children
Toronto, Ontario, Canada
Email: sgordon@sickkids.ca
Chapter 4

Fumio Hanaoka
Graduate School of Frontier Biosciences
SORST
Japan Science and Technology
　Corporation
Suita, Osaka, Japan
Preface

Laura S. Haneline
Department of Pediatrics
Herman B. Wells Center
　for Pediatric Research
Indianapolis, Indiana, U.S.A.
Email: lhanelin@iupui.edu
Chapter 3

Gary M. Kupfer
Department of Microbiology
Department of Pediatrics
Division of Pediatric
  Hematology-Oncology
University of Virginia
Charlottesville, Virginia, U.S.A.
Email: gk9e@virginia.edu
Chapter 6

Johnson M. Liu
Schneider Children's Hospital
Pediatric Hematology/Oncology
  and Stem Cell Transplantation
New Hyde Park, New York, U.S.A.
Email: jliu3@NSHS.edu
Chapter 8

Tetsuya Otsuki
Clinical Science Planning
  and Development
Banyu (Merck-Japan) Pharmaceutical
  Company
Tokyo, Japan
Email: tetsuya_otsuki@merck.com
Chapter 8

Giovanni Pagano
Centre for Research
Innovation and Technology Transfer
  in Oncology and Life Sciences
Mercogliano (AV), Italy
Email: gbpagano@tin.it
Chapter 9

Filippo Rosselli
Laboratory of Genetic Stability
  and Cancer
UPR 2169, CNRS
Gustave Roussy Institute PR2
Villejuif, France
Email: Rosselli@igr.fr
Chapter 5

Akira Tachibana
Radiation Biology Center
Kyoto University
Kyoto, Japan
Email:
  atachibana@house.rbc.kyoto_u.ac.jp
Chapter 11

A. Malcolm R. Taylor
CR-UK Institute for Cancer Studies
University of Birmingham
Birmingham, England, U.K.
Email: A.M.R.Taylor@bham.ac.uk
Chapter 1

Takayuki Yamashita
Division of Genetic Diagnosis
Institute of Medical Science
University of Tokyo
Tokyo, Japan
Email: y-taka@showa.gunma-u.ac.jp
Chapter 7

PREFACE

Fanconi anemia (FA) is a rare largely autosomal recessive genetic disorder (one complementation group being X-linked) that was first recognized almost 40 years ago[5] as a cause of juvenile leukemia. Other phenotypes include bone marrow failure leading to aplastic anemia, growth retardation, congenital malformations of renal, cardiac, skeletal and skin structures, pancytopenia and pronounced cancer predisposition.

Interestingly FA shares a number of clinical and molecular features with a variety of other syndromes, including Seckel syndrome[1] and Nijmegen breakage syndrome,[6] and further investigation of all three conditions will provide insights into the molecular mechanisms involved in each one and where they may interact.

In the recent past much effort has gone into understanding the molecular pathogenesis of FA in terms of enhanced susceptibility to DNA damaging agents. Results of these studies have yielded exciting information on a multiplicity of hitherto unknown protein-protein interactions involved in activities from control of redox state and apoptosis to repair of DNA strand breaks.[15]

Working with the leading researchers and clinicians in the field, this book has been produced to provide a comprehensive treatise on FA. This covers in detail what is known of the 12 complementation groups identified to date. These include FANCA, -B (X-linked, localized at Xp22.31),[11] -C, -D1, -D2, -E, -F, -G, -I, -J, -L and M.

There is clear variation in the clinical features exhibited by sufferers in different complementation groups, and even between those with different mutations of the same gene. This is explored in detail in Chapter 1 and expanded upon in the introduction to Chapter 5. The link between mutation and phenotype may ultimately help pick apart the complex cellular actions of the FANC proteins. At the other end of the spectrum and the book, Chapter 10 details the best treatments as currently perceived for FA. Whilst the future holds out the possibility of gene therapy or protein replacement, the treatment of choice at present is still stem cell or bone marrow transplantation from a matched sibling.[7,8]

Chapter 3 introduces the *FANC* genes identified to date and their products. It is apparent that FANCA, -B,-C,-E, -F, -G and -L form a core complex within the nucleus of cells leading to monoubiquitination of FANCD2. ATR checkpoint kinase and RPA1 are required for efficient FANCD2 monoubiquitination.[1] The nature and roles of this complex are the subjects of Chapter 7. FANCD1 and FANCJ appear to act downstream, being actively recruited along with BRCA1 and RAD51 to chromatin at specific foci for the repair of DNA damage. The precise role of FANCI has not yet been determined but it seems to act at a stage between core complex formation and FANCD2 ubiquitination.[10] The involvement of breast cancer susceptibility and FA genes in this pathway is an area of active research. It is evident that FA-D1 patients are predisposed to breast cancer,[16] although members of the other FA complementation groups do not show a high frequency of this malignancy.[14] This would seem to indicate that the BRCA proteins may exert their breast cancer preventative function independently of FANCD2 ubiquitination (although see below). BRCA1 and BRCA2 are known to be independently involved in other activities including regulation of differentiation, and it may be that the disruption of these impacts on breast cancer development.[9]

In addition to their central role in DNA repair the FA proteins are intimately involved in a range of other cellular functions through their individual interactions with other proteins. This concept is introduced in Chapter 2 where proteins interacting with FANCA, FANCC and FANCG are introduced. Several of these interactions are with proteins involved in maintenance of redox balance. In Chapter 9, Pagano and Ahmad, long term proponents of the oxidative stress theory of FA, expand upon the ways in which interruptions in FA-redox protein associations could result in the phenotypic abnormalities observed in FA, providing an alternative model to the more widely accepted DNA repair deficiency. Abnormalities in mitochondrial function in FA further support a role of oxidative stress.[4] It is likely that it is a combination of a deficiency in redox control and ineffective DNA repair which give the complex clinical characteristics of this disorder: many of the congenital abnormalities arising due to the former, and predisposition to malignancy to the latter. It is highly probable, however, that the debate over the relative contributions of these two phenomena will continue for some time.

Mutations in FANCA, -C and -G are the most prevalent and the individual genes and their products are considered in detail in Chapters 3-5. Interestingly other proteins which FANCA, -C and -G interact with are known or suggested to be involved in chromatin remodeling (e.g., FAZF[13] and BRG1),[12] and FANCC in particular appears to have a role in protection against cytokine-induced apoptosis in haematopoietic cells. These phenomena are discussed in detail in Chapters 4 and 8 and evidence is beginning to appear to suggest that different structural domain within FANCC are responsible for its different activities. FANCG contains sequence motifs typical of a protein involved in protein-protein interactions, and it is essential for the functional interaction between FANCC and FANCA. In turn its ability to interact with FANCA requires the presence of FANCB, -C and -F, illustrating further the intricate interplay of these proteins which is explored in detail in Chapter 5.

Chapter 6 considers the natures of FANCD1 and -D2 proteins. The exciting discovery that FANCD1 is in fact the breast cancer susceptibility gene product BRCA2, and that ubiquitinated FANCD2 interacts with BRCA1 have hugely expanded the research efforts in this area. The nuclear FA complex appears to exert its effects in a two pronged approach: by ubiquitination of FANCD2 which in turn recruits BRCA1 to the nuclear foci formed at DNA repair sites, and via interactions (possibly through FANCG association) with BRCA2 and RAD51, these proteins also being recruited to damage foci although seemingly independently of BRCA1.[17] The detail of these interactions and their roles in damage repair are under intense investigation, particularly as BRCA1 recruitment seems to be implicated in a range of DNA repair mechanisms.[15]

The final chapter (Chapter 12) is devoted to an in depth discussion of the mutations found in a geographically and genetically isolated Japanese FA population. Interestingly this group shows a preponderance of mutations in FANCA as is observed in the West, but also shows a higher frequency of FANCG involvement, confirming the central role of FANCA and the FANCA-FANCC-FANCG complex in protection against FA.

A recent Tunisian study of 41 families has revealed that 92% belong to the FANCA complementation group.[2] Others have identified Spanish Gypsies as the ethnic group with the world's highest prevalence of FA—the carrier frequency being 1/64-1/70.[3] Affected individuals are homozygous for a specific FANCA mutation (295C>T) leading to FANCA truncation. This mutation was not found in other Gypsy patients from Hungary, Germany, Slovakia and Ireland. In a Southern African population (South Africa, Swaziland, Mozambique and Malawi) a particular deletion mutation in FANCG (c.637 643delTAACCGCC) has been reported in 82% of FA patients. Birth incidence of FA in this population is greater than 1/40,000 which is above average in general populations. These studies are clearly indicative of founder mutation in the Spanish gypsy and Southern African populations.

There is no evidence that interest in FA is waning, and this book should provide both the experts and novice researchers in the field with an excellent overview of the current status of research and pointers to future research goals.

Note Added in Proof

In a recent study Meetei et al have identified a new complementation group, FANCM. The protein, FAAp250, is a part of the FA protein complex involving BRCA1 and BRCA2 and has sequence similarity to other known DNA repair proteins, including Hef in archaea, MPH1 in yeast and ERCC4 or XPF in human. FANCM is essential for monoubiquitination of FANCD2 and is hyperphosphorylated when DNA is damaged.

Shamim I. Ahmad, Fumio Hanaoka and Sandra H. Kirk

References

1. Andreassen PR, D'Andrea AD, Taniguchi T. ATR couples FANCD2 monoubiquitination to the DNA-damage response Genes Dev 2004; 18:1958-1963.
2. Bouchlaka C, Abdelhak S, Dellagi K. Molecular study of Fanconi anemia in Tunisia. Tunisia Med 2004; 82:4023-410
3. Callen E, Cassado JA, Tischkowitz MD et al. A common founder mutation in FANCA underlies the world highest prevalence of Fanconi anemia in gypsy families in Spain. Blood 2005; 105:1946-1949.
4. Clarke AA, Gibson FM, Scott J et al. Fanconi anemia cell lines show distinct mechanisms of cell death in response to mitomycin C or agonistic anti-Fas antibodies. Haematologica 2004; 89:11-20
5. Fanconi G. Familial constitutional panmyelocytopathy, Fanconi's anemia (FA). I Clinical aspects. Semin Hematol 1967; 4:233
6. Gennery AR, Slatter MA, Bhattacharya A et al. The clinical and biological overlap between Nijmegen breakage syndrome and Fanconi anemia. Clin Immunol 2004; 113:214-219.
7. Grewal SS, Kahn JP, McMillan ML et al. Successful haematopoietic stem cell transplantation for Fanconi anemia from an unaffected HLA-genotype-identical sibling selected using preimplantation genetic diagnosis. Blood 2004; 103:1147-1151
8. Guardiola P, Socie G, Li X et al. Acute graft versus-host disease in patients with Fanconi anemia or acquired aplastic anemia undergoing bone marrow transplantation from HLA-identical sibling donors: Risk factors and influence on outcome. Blood 2003; 103:73-77
9. Kubista M, Rosner M, Miloloza A et al. BRCA1 and differentiation. Mut Res 2002; 512:165-172.
10. Levitus M, Rooimans MA, Steltenpool J et al. Heterogeneity in Fanconi anemia: evidence of two new genetic subtypes. Blood 2004; 103:2498-2503.
11. Meetei AR, Levitus M, Xue Y et al. X-linked inheritance of Fanconi anemia complementation group B. Nat Genet 2004; 36:1219-1224.
12. Otsuki T, Furukawa Y, Ikeda K et al. Fanconi anemia protein, FANCA associates with BRG1, a component of the human SW1/SNF complex. Hum Mol Genet 2001; 10:2651-2660.
13. Reuter TY, Medhurst AL, Waisfisz Q et al. Yeast-two hybrid screens imply involvement of Fanconi anemia proteins in transcription regulation, cell signaling, oxidative, metabolism, and cellular transport. Exp Cell Res 2003; 289:211-221.
14. Seal S, Barfoot R, Jayatilake H et al. Breast cancer susceptibility collaboration. Evaluation of Fanconi anemia genes in familial breast cancer predisposition. Cancer Res 2003; 63:8596-8599.

15. Thompson LH, Hinz JM, Yamada NA et al. How Fanconi anemia proteins promote the four RS: replication, recombination, repair and recovery. Environ Molec Mutagen 2005; 45:128-142
16. Wagner JE, Tolar J, Levran O et al. Germline mutations in BRCA2: shared genetic susceptibility to breast cancer, early onset leukemia, and Fanconi anemia. Blood 2004; 103:3226-3229.
17. Wang X, Andreassen PR, D'Andrea AD. Functional interaction of monoubiquitinated FANCD2 and BRCA2/FANCD1 in chromatin. Mol Cell Biol 2004; 24:5850-5862.
18. Meetei AR, Medhurst AL, Ling C et al. A human ortholog of archaeal DNA repair protein Hef is defective in Fanconi anemia complementation group M. Nat Genet 2005; 37:958-963.

Acknowledgments

We would like to acknowledge the continuing support of Professor Fumio Hanaoka of the University of Osaka for his encouragement in our interest in Fanconi anemia.

CHAPTER 1

Clinical Features of Fanconi Anaemia

A. Malcolm R. Taylor*

Abstract

Fanconi anaemia is an autosomal recessive disorder in which patients develop bone marrow failure and aplastic anaemia but this can occur at widely differing ages from the first year to age 12 years or more. This means that often the diagnosis is made before the onset of any haematological abnormality is apparent. Many, but not all, FA patients have quite severe congenital abnormalities and so the unusual sensitivity of FA peripheral blood lymphocytes to DNA crosslinking agents has been an important part of the diagnosis in FA. FA patients, however, may have neither bone marrow failure nor congenital abnormalities, when a diagnosis of FA is suspected and this has led to occasional confusion with Nijmegen Breakage syndrome where there is also unusual sensitivity to DNA crosslinking agents. In contrast cells from FA patients, with some rare exceptions, do not show an increased sensitivity to ionising radiation. The absence of particular FANC proteins can result in a more severe phenotype; for example the predisposition to both the presence of congenital abnormalities with early diagnosis in patients with *FANCD2* mutations and very early onset of myeloid or lymphoid leukaemia as well as carcinomas in the case of patients with *FANCD1* mutations. The pathogenesis of bone marrow failure and congenital abnormalities is not understood in the context of the loss of particular FANC proteins. In addition, the number of genes identified is fairly large and their exact roles in the FA pathways have not yet been fully worked out. Although the cellular targets for these different FA proteins and the FA pathway have not yet been elucidated there appears to be a role for the FA proteins in homology directed repair of DNA double strand breaks.

Introduction

The interest in the autosomal recessive disorders Fanconi anaemia (FA), Ataxia-telangiectasia (A-T), and Bloom syndrome (BS) was originally driven by the knowledge that each group of patients has a strong predisposition to cancer, with a different spectrum of tumours in each disorder.[1] In addition, it had been shown that spontaneously occurring chromosome abnormalities occurred in FA, A-T and BS and they became known as the Chromosome Instability Syndromes. Although this title perhaps inferred something similar about the chromosome abnormality between them it was, in fact, quite different in each disorder. The notion that the chromosome abnormality was related to the tumour predisposition was clearly suspected although the mechanism for this, in each case, was not then understood. Patients with another disorder, Xeroderma pigmentosum (XP) who have a predisposition to skin cancer were first shown to be unusually sensitive to an environmental agent, ultraviolet light (UV).[2] This was demonstrated to be the result of a defect in DNA excision repair of UV induced pyrimidine dimers. Thereafter, FA and A-T patients were shown to be unusually sensitive to DNA

*A. Malcolm R. Taylor—CR-UK Institute for Cancer Studies, University of Birmingham, Vincent Drive, Edgbaston, Birmingham B15 2TT, England, U.K. Email: A.M.R.Taylor@bham.ac.uk

Molecular Mechanisms of Fanconi Anemia, edited by Shamim I. Ahmad and Sandra H. Kirk.
©2006 Eurekah.com and Springer Science+Business Media.

crosslinking agents, mitomycin C (MMC) and diepoxybutane (DEB)[3] and ionising radiation[4] respectively, with the inference that they also would have a defect in some form of DNA repair. Subsequently another group of patients, with Nijmegen Breakage Syndrome (NBS),[5] were described with spontaneous chromosome abnormalities like those of A-T, an unusual sensitivity to ionising radiation[6] and a predisposition to lymphoid tumours,[7] again like A-T. The various genes for XP (XPA-G and variant) and also those for A-T (*ATM* and *hMRE11*),[8-10] NBS (*NBS1*)[11,12] and BS (*BLM*) were identified and the molecular pathology of each of these disorders has been investigated intensively since. In contrast to A-T and BS, but in this respect more similar to XP, several genes have been identified that, when mutated, give rise to FA. A relationship has been demonstrated between FA, A-T[13] and disorders where either *hMRE11* or *NBS1* are mutated.[14] Therefore, interestingly, there has been some convergence of these disorders or at least the biochemical pathways underlying them and they have now been referred to as genomic instability syndromes.[15]

Genetics of Fanconi Anaemia

There are 12 different complementation groups for Fanconi anaemia of which nine, *FANCA*, *FANCB*, *FANCC*, *FANCD1*(*BRCA2*), *FANCD2*, *FANCE*, *FANCF*, *FANCG* (*XRCC9*) *FANCL* and *FANCM* have been cloned. Genes for FANCI, FANCJ remain to be cloned. The FA genes are quite different from each other showing little or no homology.

The proteins encoded by *FANCA*, *FANCC*, *FANCE*, *FANCF*, *FANCG* (*XRCC9*) and *FANCL* form a nuclear complex that acts as a ubiquitin ligase with the FANCL component being the catalytic subunit.[16] The protein complex is required for the damage induced monoubiquitination of the downstream FANCD2 protein (see also the section below on confirmation of the diagnosis of FA). The monoubiquitinated (activated) form of FANCD2 colocalises with BRCA1,[13] BRCA2 (FANCD1)[17] and NBS[14] in nuclear foci as part of the response to DNA damage. FANCI may also be part of this complex.[18] Recently, following an analysis of this same protein complex, Meetei et al[19] identified a protein they termed FAAP95 encoded by a gene on the X chromosome. They were able to show that knockdown of this protein resulted in reduced ubiquitination of FANCD2. Further, they showed that *FAAP95* mutations are the likely cause of FA-B. FANCD2 can be monoubiquitinated in both FANCD1/BRCA2 and FA-J cells[18] indicating that both FANCD1 and the predicted FANCJ protein act downstream in the FA pathway.

A surprising and intriguing finding was that the FA-D1 complementation group results from biallelic mutation of *BRCA2*,[20] mutation of which is associated with predisposition to breast and other cancers. The BRCA2 protein has known functions in homologous recombination repair.[21] Although biallelic null mutations in mice are embryonic lethal *FANCD1* Fanconi patients have hypomorphic alleles resulting in expression of some truncated BRCA2 with partial activity (see below for characteristics of FA-D1 patients).

Since FA patients' cells are unusually sensitive to DNA crosslinking agents it is presumed that a role of the FA protein complex is the resolution of DNA crosslinks. Interestingly, however, relatively little has been done on this repair pathway. The targets of the FA pathway are not presently known. Overall, the normal function of the FA/BRCA1/2 pathway is assumed to be part of the cellular response to damage present at S phase as a consequence of DNA interstrand crosslinks. Monoubiquitinated FANCD2 is required for targeting BRCA2 to chromatin.[17] Given the involvement of FANCD1(BRCA2) in homologous recombination repair these results suggests that the FA protein complex, generally, is also involved in this pathway. Indeed, both upstream FANCA and FANCG and downstream—FANCD2—proteins appear to be involved in repair of homology directed repair of DNA double strand break (DSB) and also single strand annealing.[22]

Table 1. Clinical features of Fanconi anaemia

Present at birth
- Microcephaly
- Growth retardation
- Skin pigmentation abnormalities
- Congenital abnormalities
  - Upper limb abnormalities (thumb and radial ray abnormalities)
  - Renal
  - Urogenital
  - Gastrointestinal
  - Other
- Neurological

Variable age of onset
- Bone marrow failure
- Myelodysplastic syndrome (MDS)
- Acute myeloid leukaemia (AML)
- Carcinomas

Adapted from data in Duckworth–Rysiecki et al, 1984;[42] Alter, 1993;[38] Faivre et al, 2000;[39] Tischkowitz and Hodgson, 2003;[35] Huber and Mathew, 2004[41]

Clinical Features of Fanconi Anaemia (Table 1)

FA is a rare disorder with an incidence of approximately 3 cases per million,[23,24] very similar to the birth frequency of A-T.[25] The median survival period is ~24 years.[26] Since so many genes are now known to be involved in the development of FA a considerable degree of clinical heterogeneity might be predicted, although the degree of heterogeneity may also depend on the frequency of each genotype.

Haematological Abnormalities

This is the most serious and consistent of the clinical features of FA.[27] In the original publication by Fanconi (1927) the aplastic anaemia was the major finding in the report on the three affected brothers. It would seem appropriate, therefore that a *sine qua non* for the diagnosis of FA would be the presence of aplastic anaemia. The problem is that the pancytopenia is not usually present at birth but only develops later, in most instances between the ages of 5 and 10 years with median age of onset at 7 years.[28] However, other features of FA, like the presence of congenital abnormalities, may be immediately apparent and diagnosis is frequently made before the onset of the aplastic anaemia. This can have the advantage that, if the diagnosis is correctly made, the eventual anaemia may be better managed. Exceptionally, pancytopenia is seen as early as neonatal life and Landmann et al[29] reported pancytopenia at age 2 weeks in a FA patient without congenital abnormalities with the homozygous *FANCG* mutation 1649delC.

Bone marrow failure precedes the development of myelodysplastic syndrome (MDS) or acute myeloid leukaemia (AML) although occasionally patients can present with either of these. Drawing on data from three sources, a literature survey,[30] the North American Survey of 145 Fanconi patients[31] and the International Fanconi Anaemia Registry (IFAR) study,[26] Alter et al[32] suggested that the cumulative incidence of any haematological finding in FA may be as high as 90%, and bone marrow failure requiring therapy was ~60%. This agrees with an earlier estimate by the International Fanconi Anaemia Registry[33] that the actuarial risk of developing any haematopoietic abnormality by age 40 was 98%; the risk of pancytopenia was 84% by the age of 20 years and the risk of either MDS or AML was about 50% by age 40 years (MDS and AML were not considered separately). Death resulted from haematological causes in 80% of cases by age 40 years. The risk of bone marrow failure was highest in patients with abnormal

Table 2. Malignant disease in Fanconi anaemia patients

Leukaemias
    Acute myeloid leukaemia (AML) – 5-10% risk
    Myelodysplatic syndrome – ~5% risk
    Acute T cell leukaemia (T-ALL) – rare; only reported in FANCD1(BRCA2) patients
Carcinomas
    Liver tumours – may be related to treatment
    Head and neck tumours
    Oesophagus
    Vulva
Embryonal tumours
    Wilms tumour – rare; only reported in FANCD1(BRCA2) patients
Brain tumours
    Medulloblastoma – rare; only reported in FANCD1(BRCA2) patients
    Astrocytoma – rare; only reported in FANCD1(BRCA2) patients

Adapted from data in Offit et al, 2003;[56] Hirsch et al, 2004;[55] Wagner et al, 2004;[30] Alter, 2003;[28] Alter et al, 2003[32]

radii and a 5-point congenital abnormality score.[34] Conversely the greatest risk for developing AML or a solid tumour occurred in the longest lived patients – those with the lowest risk of bone marrow failure.[34]

Approximately 30% of FA patients studied by Rosenberg et al[31] and Kutler et al[26] received a bone marrow transplant (BMT). In the 145 patients in the study of Rosenberg et al[31] 44 patients underwent BMT, 37 for aplastic anaemia and 7 for MDS. The complications of BMT also carry a risk of death.[33,35]

Leukaemia in Fanconi Anaemia

According to Alter et al[32] the individual's risk of MDS was ~5% with the evolution to AML not being inevitable. Their estimate was that, in addition, there was a 5-10% individual risk of AML in FA.

Solid Tumours (Table 2)

The risk of solid tumours increases with age with the risk being 5-10% and cumulative risk of ~30% by age 45 years,[32] greater than for AML. Young adults with FA show an increased risk of head and neck squamous cell carcinomas tumours, tumours of oesophagus, kidney (including embryonic Wilms tumours and nephroblastoma – see below), brain (mainly medulloblastoma), liver, vulva and cervix. The occurrence of liver tumours may be related to treatment with androgens (oxymethalone) for bone marrow failure. Some patients have also developed two tumours and, more rarely, more than two.[26] The conditioning regimen for BMT is also associated with risk of induction of malignant disease. The risk of squamous cell carcinomas of the head, neck and oesophagus was reportedly higher in FA patients who had received a bone marrow transplant and occurred at an earlier age than nontransplanted patients.[36]

Presenting Features of FA (Table 1)

Small stature and the presence of one or more congenital abnormalities (principally microcephaly and abnormalities of skin pigmentation) in the absence of aplastic anaemia is, therefore, how many FA patients present. They show slower growth both in utero, with lower birth weight, and after birth. This may be further complicated by the presence of hormonal deficiencies.[35,37] Two thirds of patients will also show multiple congenital abnormalities. These include upper limb abnormalities, especially absent radius and thumb anomalies, as well as renal abnormalities (e.g., horseshoe kidney). Less commonly there may be abnormalities of the urogenital and gastrointestinal systems, the lower limbs, cardiopulmonary defects, deafness and neurological abnormalities[38,39] as well as more rare pathologies.[40]

The major method for laboratory confirmation of the presence of FA has been to use a peripheral blood sample to demonstrate the unusual chromosomal sensitivity of FA patients' cells to DNA crosslinking agents (see ref. 41). Cells from all FA patients show increased sensitivity to DNA crosslinking agents although there is some variation between patients in the level of induced damage. The level of spontaneously occurring chromosome damage is variable being raised in lymphocytes from many but not all FA patients.[42]

Fanconi Anaemia and Nijmegen Breakage Syndrome

Not all FA patients show the presence of congenital skeletal, gastrointestinal, renal tract or central nervous system (CNS) abnormalities. Indeed a study suggested that as many as a third of patients fall into this category.[43] If a diagnosis of FA anaemia is suspected at an early age in this group of patients, the aplastic anaemia is unlikely to be present and the diagnosis relies on the presence of other features such as microcephaly, growth retardation and abnormalities of skin pigmentation.

NBS patients also share some features with FA including microcephaly and skin pigmentation changes (Table 3). Recently, a patient originally diagnosed at age 2 years with atypical FA was shown to be homozygous for an *NBS1* mutation (*NBS1* 1089C>A; Y363X which is different from the common 657del5 Slavic mutation) and showed total cellular loss of Nbs1 protein.[14,44] The patient did not show any aplastic anaemia, but did show microcephaly, skin pigmentation abnormalities, thrombocytosis, mild lymphopaenia, recurrent upper respiratory tract infections with an increased level of DEB induced chromosome breakage and so was classed as having FA.[44] This patient had two siblings with the same symptoms and a diagnosis of FA was again made on the basis of these features and a positive DEB test. Their cousin, patient 1,[44] showed microcephaly, failure to thrive, recurrent chest infections, and *café au lait* spots. Later immunodeficiency was also diagnosed. She subsequently developed a plasma cell tumour and died. None of these patients had developed an aplastic anaemia but a second child of ~4 years died from complications following an infection and two patients aged ~6 and 3 years, respectively, are alive.

Cells from both A-T like disorder (ATLD- mutated for hMRE11) and NBS patients have also been shown to be unusually sensitive to DNA crosslinking agents, DEB and MMC.[14] This observation, therefore, showed that increased sensitivity to either of these agents is not specific for FA.

A further report[45] described two patients in two related families where FA was a possible diagnosis but in fact the patients were shown to have the *NBS1* 1089C>A; Y363X mutation and apparent total absence of Nbs1. Interestingly, this is the same mutation as the patients described above.[14,44] The patients described by Gennery et al[45] were small with microcephaly, repeated infections, immunodeficiency and failure to thrive. Radial ray anomalies and aplastic anaemia were not present. The authors suggested that the clinical features of these NBS patients appeared to be particularly severe compared with other NBS patients. It is not clear how the *NBS1* 1089C>A; Y363X homozygous mutation results in this particular phenotype. Although full length Nbs1 protein could not be demonstrated, it is unlikely to be totally absent as most NBS patients show some truncated Nbs1 and total absence of the protein is embryonic lethal in mice.

In conclusion, cells from these patients show that (i) increased sensitivity to DNA crosslinking agents like MMC and DEB is not specific to FA patients and indeed it is common to patients with FA, NBS and ATLD as well as cells from some Seckel syndrome patients[46] (ii) in the absence of congenital abnormalities, there is some overlap of clinical features between FA and NBS especially with regard to microcephaly and skin changes although the primary immunodeficiency of NBS is not seen in FA and aplastic anaemia associated with FA is not seen in NBS.

Table 3. Comparison of features of Fanconi anaemia and Nijmegen Breakage syndrome

Feature	Fanconi Anaemia	Nijmegen BS
CLINICAL		
Microcephaly	yes	yes
Growth retardation	yes	yes
Skin pigmentation abnormalities	yes	yes
Typical facies	yes (some)	yes
Craniofacial features	yes (some)	yes (all)
Learning difficulties	minority	majority
Aplastic anaemia	yes (later onset)	no
Primary immunodeficiency	no	yes
Infections	no	yes
Myeloid tumours	yes	no
Lymphoid tumours	rare	yes
Other tumours	yes (carcinomas)	yes (no carcinomas)
Congenital Abnormalities	yes	minor or rare
Radial ray abnormalities	yes	no
Renal abnormalities	yes	no
Urogenital abnormalities	yes	no
Deafness	yes	no
CYTOGENETICS OF PERIPHERAL LYMPHOCYTES		
Spontaneous random breakage	yes (some)	no (low)
Translocations t(7;14) etc	no	yes
CELLULAR		
Increased sensitivity to		
DNA cross linking agents	yes	yes
Ionising radiation	no (rare exceptions)	yes (all)

Adapted from data in Hiel et al, 2000;[7] Alter, 1993;[30] Faivre et al, 2000;[39] Tischkowitz and Hodgson, 2003;[35] Huber and Mathew, 2004[41]

Confirmation of the Diagnosis in FA Patients

The finding that increased sensitivity to either MMC or DEB is not specific for FA has influenced the methods of confirmation of the diagnosis. However, where there is both aplastic anaemia and congenital abnormalities, FA is a likely diagnosis. In this group of patients, the presence of increased chromosome breakage, following exposure of blood to DNA crosslinking agents, should confirm the diagnosis. The majority of FA patients are in complementation groups FANCA (~70%), FANCC (~10%) and FANCG (~10%). Complementation analysis by infection with retrovirus containing a cDNA from a FA gene[47] will identify the particular FANC gene and subsequent DNA sequencing will identify the gene mutation in the vast majority of these cases.

An alternative method for establishing the likelihood that a patient has FA is to examine the ability of the patient's primary lymphocytes to monoubiquitinate the FANCD2 protein.[13,16,47] The FANCA, FANCC, FANCE, FANCF, FANCG and FANCL proteins interact with each other and the complex is required for the monoubiquitination of the downstream protein FANCD2. Protein extracts of normal cells immunoblotted for FANCD2 show two bands, with the larger form being the ubiquitinated FANCD2. Cells from FA patients with mutations in FANCA, FANCC, FANCE, FANCF, FANCG or FANCL express only the nonubiquitinated smaller isoform of FANCD2. The absence of the ubiquitinated band in cell extract from a patient will indicate FA caused by mutation in one of these genes. This of course will be the majority of FA patients. Complementation analysis, followed by sequencing, will identify the FANC gene mutation. Some caution is required as there are other FANC genes. The very rare *FANCD1(BRCA2)* mutation encodes a protein that functions downstream of FANCD2 and so ubiquitination of FANCD2 in cells from such a patient will give a false negative result.

In addition, mosaicism in blood cells may also lead to a false negative if the revertant normal population is large enough. Mosaicism for cells with either biallelic or single FANC mutations affects a minority of FA individuals and seen as a clear unusual sensitivity to the chromosome damaging effects of crosslinking agents in some blood lymphocytes but not in others. Recently, Soulier et al[48] reported the presence of mosaicism as shown by the presence of a light monoubiquitinated FANCD2 band in FA-A peripheral blood cells. What is the mechanism for the reversion of phenotype? Reversion of a mutation in cells heterozygous for a mutation may occur through gene conversion. In the case of FA, where both alleles are mutant, one mechanism, for example, was described in which a single base deletion (resulting in a frameshift mutation) was compensated by two additional single base deletions resulting in expression of some functional protein.[49]

The presence of aplastic anaemia cannot be an absolute requirement for a clinical diagnosis of FA because of it relatively late onset in childhood in most cases. In the absence, therefore, of congenital abnormalities as well as aplastic anaemia an increased sensitivity to DNA crosslinking agents could also be an indication that the patient might have NBS. Laboratory features of NBS should be investigated including, definitively, the identification of *NBS1* mutations. In addition, loss of full length Nbs1 protein by Western blotting, a substantially increased sensitivity to ionizing radiation and the presence of translocations involving chromosomes 7 and 14 in the peripheral blood can also be examined.

Relationship of Complementation Group to Clinical Features

It is unclear how much correlation exists between a FA complementation group and clinical findings. Different interacting factors will affect any putative correlation. (1) Bearing in mind the fact that many of the FANC proteins contribute to a single core complex, which activates FANCD2 by monoubiquitination, it is possible that loss of any one of these proteins may have the same effect of destabilising the complex. The inference of this may be that the clinical features associated with loss of any one component of the complex may be similar. Of course, it is possible that individual components of the complex may have functions in addition to those of the core complex. This might lead to gene specific phenotypes. (2) FA-A patients are the largest group and mutation specific effects (e.g., the presence of a particular missense mutation allowing expression of some mutant FANC protein with some activity) may occur to give significant phenotypic variation within the group. (3) It is quite likely that genetic background or modifying genes will also contribute to the effects of particular FA mutations. This may be more readily observed for the numerically larger complementation group A. (4) Finally, loss of FA proteins FANCD1(BRCA2), FANCD2 and the putative FANCJ that are not part of the FA protein core complex might be the ones expected to each give a consistent and different phenotype to the others.

Comparison of Patients in Complementation Groups FA-A, FA-C and FA-G (Table 4)

Some comparison can be made between these three groups because they are common enough to allow the accumulation of the numbers of patients required. It was suggested that FA-C, compared with FA-A and FA-G patients, had a significantly earlier onset of bone marrow failure and poorer survival but there was no difference in the cumulative incidence of AML and MDS between FA complementation groups A, C and G.[26] There was also poorer overall survival for patients with at least one intron 4 (*FANCC* IVS4+4A>T mutation – a founder mutation in the Jewish population)[26,50] or one *FANCC* exon 14 (R548X or L554P) mutation.[26]

Table 4. Features of patients in different complementation groups

	Frequency (%)	Specific Clinical Features	Tumours	References
Upstream				
FA-A	60-65	Mutation specific poorer survival	AML carcinomas	Kutler et al, 2003 Hermsen, 2001
FA-B	rare	NK	NK	
FA-C	10-15	Mutation specific poorer survival	AML carcinomas	Kutler et al, 2003 Hermsen, 2001
FA-E	rare	more congenital abs CNS Abs.	?	Faivre et al, 2000
FA-F	rare	more congenital Abs	NK	Faivre et al, 2000
FA-G	~10	earliery BM failure Carcinomas	AML	Kutler et al, 2003 Faivre et al, 2000
FA-I	rare	NK	NK	Levitus et al, 2004
Downstream				
FA-J	rare	NK	NK	Levitus et al, 2004
FA-D1(BRCA2)	rare	more severe (tumours early)	AML/T-ALL/Wilms Medulloblastoma	Offit et al, 2003 Hirsch et al, 2003 Wagner et al, 2003
FA-D2	rare	more severe (congenital abnormalities)	NK	Soulier et al, 2004

In contrast, however, Faivre et al[39] reporting on European FA patients, suggested that there was no difference among FA-A, FA-C and FA-G patients for age of onset of haematological abnormalities although the cytopaenia was significantly worse in FA-G. Faivre et al[39] also reported that FA-G had a higher rate of AML or MDS than FA-A or FA-C. There was a reduced incidence of congenital abnormalities in FA-C patients, excluding those with the *FANCC* IVS4+4A>T mutation, than either FA-A or FA-G, that were similar. More congenital abnormalities were associated with the *FANCC* IVS4+4A>T mutation. In contrast, patients with the *FANCC* 322delG mutation had fewer congenital abnormalities. Patients with two null *FANCA* mutations had an earlier age of onset of haematological abnormalities and shorter survival after diagnosis compared with FA-A patients who expressed some FANCA protein. The biallelic null FA-A patients also showed a greater proportion of AML/MDS compared with FA-A patients expressing some mutated FANCA protein.[39] The FANCA proteins associated with different types of *FANCA* mutations showed different levels of complementation of MMC sensitivity, indicating that some phenotypic variation within FA-A patients may be related to the type of mutation present.[51]

Patients in the Rarer FA Complementation Groups, FA-E and FA-F (Table 4)

The difficulty with the rarer groups FA-E and FA-F is the absence of any significant numbers of patients to make a real assessment of the relationship between complementation group and clinical features. Faivre et al[39] suggested that congenital abnormalities may be more common in the FA-E and F patients. Interestingly, a significantly higher proportion (3/5) of the FA-E patients presented with CNS malformations.[39]

Patients in Complementation Groups FA-D2 and FA-J (Table 4)

Very few patients have a FANCD2 mutation. Levitus et al[18] give a proportion of 8/241 FA families in the D2 complementation group. Because FANCD2 is not a part of the FA core protein complex, but a target of it, patients with FANCD2 mutations might be different from the majority of FA patients. Soulier et al[48] gave the clinical features of a group of four FANCD2 patients diagnosed at the early ages of 0.3, 3, 2.8 and 6 years. It was suggested that they had more severe congenital abnormalities than patients in other complementation groups. The observation, by Faivre et al[39] of a higher rate of congenital abnormalities in a combined group of FA-D patients is consistent with this. One FANCD2 patient showed evidence of FA reversion.[48] Soulier et al[48] also suggested that patients mutated for the putative *FANCJ* gene, coding for another downstream protein, might also have a more severe phenotype.

Although FA cells have been examined for increased radiosensitivity this is not a common finding among FA.[52] Cells from FANCD2 patients do, however, appear to show increased radiosensitivity and have a defect in the ionising radiation inducible S phase checkpoint as do A-T cells. The ATM dependent phosphorylation of FANCD2 on serine 222 is required for activation of the radiation induced S phase checkpoint.[53] This is additional to the FA complex dependent monoubiquitination of FANCD2 on K561 as part of a second pathway in response to damage by DNA crosslinking agents. Interestingly the mouse model of *Fancd2*$^{-/-}$ mice also exhibit a more severe phenotype.[54] However, *Fancd2*$^{-/-}$ deficient mouse cells do not show an increased cellular radiosensitivity or radioresistant DNA synthesis.[54] This is different to the FANCD2 cells but the reason for this difference is not known.

Patients in Complementation Group FA-D1(Brca2) (Table 4)

It has recently become clear that FA patients with biallelic mutation of *BRCA2* have a severe phenotype, at least in terms of predisposition to early onset of cancer compared with other FA groups.[28,55,56] Two recent studies on a total of 11 patients have highlighted both the increased risk of AML (6 cases) and acute T cell leukaemia (2 cases)[28,55] and solid tumours including medulloblastoma (2 cases) and Wilms tumour (3 cases) in these patients.[55] All 11 patients developed a tumour before the age of 5 years and two patients had two tumours. Leukaemia occurred at a median age of 2.2 years compared with a median age of onset of 13.4 years in other FA patients.[28] It is clear that different tumour types can occur in the presence of the same *BRCA2* mutations; one of these patients had both Wilms tumour and T-ALL. What range of tumours will be associated with biallelic mutation of BRCA2 remains to be seen. Microcephaly, intra-uterine growth retardation, failure to thrive, short stature and *café au lait* spots were common features to these patients. Severe congenital abnormalities were largely absent and only 4 patients presented with bone marrow failure. Mutations of BRCA2 were demonstrated in all the patients and loss of full length BRCA2 protein in both the families even though one family carried the BRCA2 missense mutation 7751T>C; L2510P.[55]

Bearing in mind the consequence of loss of BRCA2 in the predisposition to some breast and other tumours it might be anticipated that the families of these FANCD1 patients might be at some additional risk of tumours. A significant family history of breast cancer was noted in 3/5 of the families,[28] although there was an apparent absence of any increase in BRCA-2 related tumours in the families studied.[55]

Another interesting feature of cells from these patients was the striking increase, compared with other FA patients, of spontaneously occurring chromosome abnormalities as well as the high level of chromosome aberrations induced by DNA crosslinking agents.[55] The presence of these spontaneous types of chromosome aberration is reminiscent of those seen in other Brca2 deficient cells.[57] The evidence suggests that *Brca2*$^{-/-}$ murine cells with the deletion of the BRCA2-carboxy terminus are hypersensitive to ionizing radiation (IR),[58-60] although it is not clear whether this is true of the human BRCA$^{-/-}$ (CAPAN-1) cells. However, the increase in the radiosensitivity does not appear to be as great as for A-T cells. Interestingly, there is no published data indicating whether or not FANCD1 cells are unusually sensitive to IR although,

Hirsch et al[55] suggest, without data being presented, that some of their FA-D1 cells show a marked sensitivity to ionising radiation. It remains unclear, therefore, whether the FA-D1 cells are indeed unusually radiosensitive. Indeed, it is not certain that this would be the case if these cells carry hypomorphic alleles of *BRCA2*.

The evidence is that BRCA2 functions in the same cellular pathway as other FA proteins and, therefore, the cause of the more severe clinical appearance of BRCA2 mutant FA patients is intriguing?

Evidence for Modifying Mutations

As expected, FA patients within a family, homozygous for the same FANC mutation, may show similar clinical phenotypes.[61] However, this is not always the case. Studying (1) the clinical variation between FA patients within other families (2) differences between families homozygous for the same FANC mutation (3) the effects of the presence of the same mutation on a different genetic background will all provide some evidence as to whether other factors play a role in the development of the FA phenotypes. In two related FA-A families with four affected children, all sharing the same homozygous deletion of *FANCA* exon 43 there was marked variation in the severity of the congenital abnormalities[62] between the two families suggesting some possible effect of genetic background. Futaki et al[63] also suggested that modifying genes or other factors contributed to the clinical phenotype since they were able to show that Japanese patients with the *FANCC* IVS4+4A>T mutation had the same severity of clinical phenotype as other Japanese FA patients with different *FANC* mutations. This contrasts with the more severe clinical phenotype associated with the *FANCC* IVS4+4A>T mutation in Ashkenazi Jewish patients.[64]

Conclusions

FA patients present with a wide range of phenotypes and it is quite possible that other rare complementation groups remain to be defined. From the data already available it seems likely that that some clear clinical differences will be established between those patients whose mutations affect the FANC protein core complex compared with those whose mutations affect the downstream proteins FANCD1 and FANCD2. A surprising finding has been the predisposition to early onset tumours of different histological type that occurs in the FANCD1 (BRCA2) patients. Particularly intriguing are reports of T cell tumours in these patients. T cell leukaemia also occurs with high frequency in patients with A-T and these observations may be an indication of a further interaction between ATM and the FANC pathway, involving FANCD1 (BRCA2). The major challenge is to define the targets of the FANC proteins, to understand the FA pathway and reexamine the clinical phenotypes in light of this knowledge.

Acknowledgements

The author thanks CR-UK, The Kay Kendall Leukaemia Fund, the Leukaemia Research Fund and the Ataxia Telangiectasia Society for continued support.

References

1. Taylor AMR. Chromosome instability syndromes. Bailliere's Best Practice & Research Clinical Haematology 2001; 14:631-644.
2. Cleaver JE. Defective repair replication of DNA in Xeroderma pigmentosum. Nature 1968; 218:652-6.
3. Sasaki MS, Tonomura A. A high susceptibility of Fancon's anaemia to chromosome breakage by DNA crosslinking agents. Cancer Res 1973; 33:1829-1836.
4. Taylor AM, Harnden DG, Arlett CF et al. Ataxia telangiectasia: A human mutation with abnormal radiation sensitivity. Nature 1975; 258:427-9.
5. Weemaes CM, Hustinx TW, Scheres JM et al. A new chromosome instability disorder: The Nijmegen breakage syndrome. 1981; 70:557-564.
6. Taalman RD, Jaspers NG, Scheres JM et al. Hypersensitivity to ionizing radiation, in vitro, in a new chromosomal breakage disorder, the Nijmegen Breakage Syndrome. Mutat Res 1983; 112:23-32.

7. Hiel JAP et al (International Nijmegen Breakage Study Group). Nijmegen breakage syndrome. The International Nijmegen Breakage Syndrome Study Group. Arch Dis Child 2000; 82:400-6.
8. Hernandez D, McConville CM, Stacey M et al. A family showing no evidence of linkage between the ataxia telangiectasia gene and chromosome 11q22-23. J Med Genet 1993; 30:135-40.
9. Savitsky K, Bar-Shira A, Gilad S et al. A single ataxia telangiectasia gene with a product similar to PI-3 kinase. Science 1995; 268:1749-53.
10. Stewart GS, Maser RS, Stankovic T et al. The DNA double-strand break repair gene hMRE11 is mutated in individuals with an ataxia-telangiectasia-like disorder. Cell 1999; 99:577-87.
11. Carney JP, Maser RS, Olivares H et al. The hMre11/hRad50 protein complex and Nijmegen breakage syndrome: Linkage of double-strand break repair to the cellular DNA damage response. Cell 1998; 93:477-86.
12. Varon R, Vissinga C, Platzer M et al. Nibrin, a novel DNA double-strand break repair protein, is mutated in Nijmegen breakage syndrome. Cell 1998; 93:467-76.
13. Garcia-Higuera I, Taniguchi T, Ganesan S et al. Interaction of the Fanconi anemia proteins and BRCA1 in a common pathway. Mol Cell 2001; 7:249-62.
14. Nakanishi K, Taniguchi T, Ranganathan V et al. Interaction of FANCD2 and NBS1 in the DNA damage response. Nat Cell Biol 2002; 4:913-20.
15. D'Andrea AD, Grompe M. The Fanconi anaemia/BRCA pathway. Nat Rev Cancer 2003; 3:23-34.
16. Meetei AR, de Winter JP, Medhurst AL et al. A novel ubiquitin ligase is deficient in Fanconi anemia. Nat Genet 2003; 35:165-70.
17. Wang X, Andreassen PR, D'Andrea AD. Functional interaction of monoubiquitinated FANCD2 and BRCA2/FANCD1 in chromatin. Mol Cell Biol 2004; 24:5850-62.
18. Levitus M, Rooimans MA, Steltenpool J et al. Heterogeneity in Fanconi anemia: Evidence for 2 new genetic subtypes. Blood 2004; 103:2498-503.
19. Meetei AR, Levitus M, Xue Y et al. X-linked inheritance of Fanconi anemia complementation group B. Nat Genet 2004; 36:1219-24.
20. Howlett NG, Taniguchi T, Olson S et al. Biallelic inactivation of BRCA2 in Fanconi anemia. Science 2002; 297:606-9.
21. Davies AA, Masson JY, McIlwraith MJ et al. Role of BRCA2 in control of the RAD51 recombination and DNA repair protein. Mol Cell 2001; 7:273-82.
22. Nakanishi K, Yang YG, Pierce AJ et al. Human Fanconi anemia monoubiquitination pathway promotes homologous DNA repair. Proc Natl Acad Sci USA 2005; 102:1110-15
23. Schroeder TM, Tilgen D, Kruger J et al. Formal genetics of Fanconi's anemia. Hum Genet 1976; 32:257-88.
24. Swift M, Sholman L, Perry M et al. Malignant neoplasms in the families of patients with ataxia-telangiectasia. Cancer Res 1976; 36:209-15.
25. Woods CG, Bundey SE, Taylor AM. Unusual features in the inheritance of ataxia telangiectasia. Hum Genet 1990; 84:555-62.
26. Kutler DI, Singh B, Satagopan J et al. A 20-year perspective on the International Fanconi Anemia Registry (IFAR). Blood 2003; 101:1249-56.
27. Tischkowitz M, Dokal I. Fanconi anaemia and leukaemia - clinical and molecular aspects. Br J Haematol 2004; 126:176-91.
28. Wagner JE, Tolar J, Levran O et al. Germline mutations in BRCA2: Shared genetic susceptibility to breast cancer, early onset leukemia, and Fanconi anemia. Blood 2004; 103:3226-9.
29. Landmann E, Bluetters-Sawatzki R, Schindler D et al. Fanconi anemia in a neonate with pancytopenia. J Pediatr 2004; 145:125-7.
30. Alter BP. Cancer in Fanconi anemia, 1927-2001. Cancer 2003; 97:425-40.
31. Rosenberg PS, Greene MH, Alter BP. Cancer incidence in persons with Fanconi anemia. Blood 2003; 101:822-6, (Erratum in: Blood. 2003;101:2136).
32. Alter BP, Greene MH, Velazquez I et al. Cancer in Fanconi anemia. Blood 2003; 101:2072.
33. Butturini A, Gale RP, Verlander PC et al. Hematologic abnormalities in Fanconi anemia: An international fanconi anemia registry study. Blood 1994; 84:1650-5.
34. Rosenberg PS, Huang Y, Alter BP. Individualized risks of first adverse events in patients with Fanconi anemia. Blood 2004; 104:350-5.
35. Tischkowitz MD, Hodgson SV. Fanconi anaemia. J Med Genet 2003; 40:1-10.
36. Rosenberg PS, Socie G, Alter BP et al. Risk of head and neck squamous cell cancer and death in patients with Fanconi anemia who did and did not receive transplants. Blood 2005; 105:67-73.
37. Wajnrajch MP, Gertner JM, Huma Z et al. Evaluation of growth and hormonal status in patients referred to the International Fanconi Anemia Registry. Pediatrics 2001; 107:744-54.
38. Alter BP. Fanconi's anaemia and its variability. Br J Haematol 1993; 85:9-14.

39. Faivre L, Guardiola P, Lewis C et al. Association of complementation group and mutation type with clinical outcome in Fanconi anemia. European Fanconi Anemia Research Group. Blood 2000; 6:4064-70.
40. Unal S, Ozbek N, Kara A et al. Five Fanconi anemia patients with unusual organ pathologies. Am J Hematol 2004; 77:50-4.
41. Huber PAJ, Mathew CG. Fanconi Anaemia. In: Eeles RA, Easton DF, Ponder BAJ, Eng C, eds. Genetic Predisposition to Cancer. 2nd ed. London: Arnold, 2004:180-192.
42. Duckworth-Rysiecki G, Hulten M, Mann J et al. Clinical and cytogenetic diversity in Fanconi's anaemia. J Med Genet 1984; 21:197-203.
43. Giampietro PF, Verlander PC, Davis JG et al. Diagnosis of Fanconi anemia in patients without congenital malformations: An international Fanconi Anemia Registry Study. Am J Med Genet 1997; 68:58-61.
44. New HV, Cale CM, Tischkowitz M et al. Nijmegen Breakage Syndrome diagnosed as Fanconi anaemia. Pediatr. Blood Cancer 2005; 44:1-6.
45. Gennery AR, Slatter MA, Bhattacharya A et al. The clinical and biological overlap between Nijmegen Breakage Syndrome and Fanconi anemia. Clin Immunol 2004; 113:214-9.
46. O'Driscoll M, Ruiz-Perez VL, Woods CG et al. A splicing mutation affecting expression of ataxia-telangiectasia and Rad3-related protein (ATR) results in Seckel syndrome. Nat Genet 2003; 33:497-501.
47. Shimamura A, de Oca RM, Svenson JL et al. A novel diagnostic screen for defects in the Fanconi anemia pathway. Blood 2002; 100:4649-54.
48. Soulier J, Leblanc T, Larghero J et al. Detection of somatic mosaicism and classification of Fanconi Anemia patients by analysis of the FA/BRCA pathway. Blood 2005; 105:1329-36.
49. Waisfisz Q, Morgan NV, Savino M et al. Spontaneous functional correction of homozygous Fanconi anaemia alleles reveals novel mechanistic basis for reverse mosaicism. Nat Genet 1999; 22:379-83.
50. Gillio AP, Verlander PC, Batish SD et al. Phenotypic consequences of mutations in the Fanconi anemia FAC gene: An International Fanconi Anemia Registry study. Blood 1997; 90:105-10.
51. Adachi D, Oda T, Yagasaki H et al. Heterogeneous activation of the Fanconi anemia pathway by patient-derived FANCA mutants. Hum Mol Genet 2002; 11:3125-34.
52. Duckworth-Rysiecki G, Taylor AM. Effects of ionizing radiation on cells from Fanconi's anemia patients. Cancer Res 1985; 45:416-20.
53. Taniguchi T, Garcia-Higuera I, Xu B et al. Convergence of the Fanconi anemia and ataxia telangiectasia signalling pathways. Cell 2002; 109:459-72.
54. Houghtaling S, Timmers C, Noll M et al. Epithelial cancer in Fanconi anemia complementation group D2 (Fancd2) knockout mice. Genes Dev 2003; 17:2021-35.
55. Hirsch B, Shimamura A, Moreau L et al. Association of biallelic BRCA2/FANCD1 mutations with spontaneous chromosomal instability and solid tumors of childhood. Blood 2004; 103:2554-9.
56. Offit K, Levran O, Mullaney B et al. Shared genetic susceptibility to breast cancer, brain tumors, and Fanconi anemia. J Natl Cancer Inst 2003; 95:1548-51.
57. Venkitaraman AR. Tracing the network connecting BRCA and Fanconi anaemia proteins. Nat Rev Cancer 2004; 4:266-76.
58. Morimatsu M, Donoho G, Hasty P. Cells deleted for Brca2 COOH terminus exhibit hypersensitivity to gamma-radiation and premature senescence. Cancer Res 1998; 58:3441-7.
59. Patel KJ, Yu VP, Lee H et al. Involvement of Brca2 in DNA repair. Mol Cell 1998; 1:347-57.
60. Yuan SS, Lee SY, Chen G et al. BRCA2 is required for ionizing radiation-induced assembly of Rad51 complex in vivo. Cancer Res 1999; 59:3547-51.
61. Tamary H, Dgany O, Toledano H et al. Molecular characterization of three novel Fanconi anemia mutations in Israeli Arabs. Eur J Haematol 2004; 72:330-5.
62. Koc A, Pronk JC, Alikasifoglu M et al. Variable pathogenicity of exon 43del (FAA) in four Fanconi anaemia patients within a consanguineous family. Br J Haematol 1999; 104:127-30.
63. Futaki M, Yamashita T, Yagasaki H et al. The IVS4 + 4 A to T mutation of the fanconi anemia gene FANCC is not associated with a severe phenotype in Japanese patients. Blood 2000; 95:1493-8.
64. Kutler DI, Auerbach AD. Fanconi anemia in Ashkenazi Jews. Fam Cancer 2004; 3:241-8.
65. Hermsen MA, Xie Y, Rooimans MA et al. Cytogenetic characteristics of oral squamous cell carcinomas in Fanconi anemia. Fam Cancer 2001; 1:39-43.
66. Wang X, D'Andrea AD. The interplay of Fanconi anemia proteins in the DNA damage response. DNA Repair (Amst) 2004; 3:1063-9.

CHAPTER 2

The Genetic Basis of Fanconi Anemia

Grover C. Bagby, Jr.*

Introduction

Seventy-five years ago, Dr. Guido Fanconi reported three siblings who exhibited both congenital defects and aplastic anemia.[1] Since then, we have learned that Fanconi anemia (FA) is a rare multigenic disorder (a prevalence of 1-5 per million[2]), that predisposes children and adults to life-threatening bone marrow failure, myelodysplasia,[3] acute nonlymphocytic leukemia (AML), and certain epithelial malignancies.[4-7] So far, the *sine qua non* of this disease is cytogenetic instability in vitro after exposure of FA cells to bifunctional alkylating agents.[8,9] Indeed, the current diagnostic test for Fanconi anemia, quantification of chromosomal breakage responses to alkylating agents, is based on this feature (reviewed in ref. 10). Classic clinical features such as growth retardation, small head size, *café-au-lait* spots, and radial ray defects can be strong diagnostic clues,[11] but FA can occur in patients without congenital defects and can be clinically ascertained in adulthood. In fact, some patients with very minimal blood count abnormalities have been identified only because they were siblings of known FA patients and were tested for that reason. Consequently, there is substantial phenotypic heterogeneity in FA and while some of it can be explained by genetic heterogeneity, certain of the clinical consequences are the result of gene-environment interactions.

Genetic Heterogeneity

Somatic cell fusion studies have defined 11 complementation groups, FA-A, B, C, D1, D2, E, F, G, L, I and J.[12] All eleven can be accounted for by mutations of a gene unique to that group and nine of the genes have been cloned[13-15] (Table 1). Some of the proteins encoded by the normal FANC genes contain domains that suggest some functions (FANCG for example has a number of tetratricopeptide [TPR] repeats[16]). However, with the exception of FANCD1, now known to be identical to BRCA2,[17] the genes and proteins they encode have no strong homologies to one another or to other known proteins.

Two recurring themes have emerged from published studies on the function of the FA proteins; (1) that they function to protect against genotoxic stress at least in part by forming complexes with each other and facilitating monoubiquitination of FANCD2, and (2) that the proteins also interact functionally with other proteins governing survival-signaling pathways.[18] While this second function of FA proteins involves formation of complexes, they are probably complexes composed of molecules not found in the so called "core FA complex" that consists of FANCA, FANCB, FANCC, FANCE, FANCF, FANCG and FANCL. In fact, as will be mentioned in more detail below, the definition of the "core complex" is undergoing some substantial revision.

*Grover C. Bagby, Jr.—OHSU Cancer Institute, Departments of Medicine and Molecular and Medical Genetics, Oregon Health and Science University, Portland, Oregon 97239, U.S.A. Email: grover@ohsu.edu

Molecular Mechanisms of Fanconi Anemia, edited by Shamim I. Ahmad and Sandra H. Kirk.
©2006 Eurekah.com and Springer Science+Business Media.

Table 1. The Fanconi anemia genes

Gene	Prevalence of Mutations in Patients with FA (%)	Chromosomal Location	Exon Number	Amino Acid Residues (kDa)
FANCA	70	16q24.3	43	1455 (163)
FANCB	1	Xp22.31	10	859(95)
FANCC	10	9q22.3	14	558 (63)
FANCD1 (BRCA2*)	1	13q12.3	27	3418 (384)
FANCD2	1	3p25.3	44	1451 (155,162)
FANCE	5	6p21.3	10	536 (60)
FANCF	2	11p15	1	374 (40)
FANCG	10	9p13	14	622 (48)
FANCL (PHF9)	1	2p16.1	11	373 (43)
FANCI	Not known	Not known	Not known	Not known
FANCJ	Not known	Not known	Not known	Not known

*Although a BRCA2 null genotype is an embryonic lethal phenotype, certain homozygous BRCA2 mutations that lead to C-terminal truncations, lead to FA of the D1 complementation group.

The *FANC* Genes

Reviewed below are selected features of each *FANC* gene and the proteins they encode. The chromosomal location and exon number of the genes and amino acid residues and molecular mass of the encoded proteins are listed in Table 1. A Fanconi Anemia Mutation Database, containing many FA mutations (but not all), is available (www.rockefeller.edu/fanconi/mutate). Currently, ascertainment of novel mutations is most often done by DHPLC analysis and sequencing of genomic DNA and cDNA. Apart from family studies, to confirm that an abnormality represents a mutation, complementation analysis (in which the wild type cDNA expressed in mutant cells corrects MMC/DEB sensitivity but the mutant cDNA does not) is most convincing. However, in light of the information now extant on key regions of FANC genes, some sequence variations (especially large deletions) can be assigned as mutations by deduction.

FANCA

Mutations of this gene are by far the most common in patients with FA, accounting for 65% of all cases. The spectrum and scope of discrete mutations of this gene are immense and include nonsense, missense, and splicing mutations as well as microdeletions, microinsertions, and duplications.[19] There may be more than 250 different mutant FANCA alleles, many of which are large intragenic deletions,[20] and only a few are common especially c.1115_1118delTTGG (2% of FANCA alleles) and c.3788_3790delTCT (5% of FANCA alleles).[19] The protein participates as a member of the core complex required for FANCD2 ubiquitination,[21] and binds to BRCA1,[22] but the functional role it plays in these complexes are unknown.

Post translational modifications of FANCA occur in response to environmental cues. For example, FANCA is redox-responsive and multimerizes with FANCG in response to oxidative stress.[23] Phosphorylation of FANCA also occurs in normal cells but not in most FA cells. In vitro phosphorylation studies identified a cytoplasmic serine kinase embedded in the core complex (sensitive to wortmannin) that phosphorylated FANCA on serines.[24] The functional consequences of this post-translational change and whether this putative FANCA kinase is the one that seems to be modulated by AKT[25] are unknown.

Like FANCC, FANCA also seems to participate directly in support of survival signal transduction pathways. For example, FANCA interacts with IKK2 and may thereby integrate with the IkappaB kinase (IKK) signalsome in a functional way. Interestingly, this IKK2 interaction is reportedly required for stimulus-dependent phosphorylation of other proteins in the FA complex.[26] FANCA also interacts with BRG1, a subunit of the SWI/SNF complex, and may regulate stress-induced chromatin remodeling.[27] Intriguingly, in FANCA mutant cells the molecular chaperone GRP94 is found in a BRG-1 associated complex but is not found in normal or complemented cells.[27] The significance of the phenomenon is unexplained but it is one of three specific examples in which aberrant or nonnative protein complexes are found in FA cells. In some instances (e.g., in the case of FANCC) there are aberrant signaling consequences that attend the formation of these complexes. Given that FANCA and FANCC both also associate with molecular chaperones,[27-29] it is quite possible that these and other FA proteins are primarily cochaperones that maintain the proper structural conformation (and state of activation or inactivation) of proteins that protect cells from environmental stresses. This theoretical model would fit with every binding phenomenon and biological function assay described to date for the FA proteins. For example, the core complex could create a scaffold for the cross-linking agent-induced activation of an ubiquitin ligase (possibly FANCL).[30]

FANCB

One of the most recently discovered FA genes was identified using a proteomics approach.[31] FANCB was discovered by mass spectrometric analysis of a 95 kDa protein found in a multimeric FA complex. It has 10 exons, 7 of which are coding exons (3-10). The C terminus of the protein contains a putative bipartite nuclear localization signal and is present in nuclear extracts of normal cells but in mutant FA-A cells, FANCB is found, like FANCL, in the cytosol. That FANCB is required for FANCD2 monoubiquitination[31] confirms that FANCB is a functional member of the core complex.

The gene encoding this protein is located at Xp22.31 and subject to X-chromosome inactivation.[31] In the cases described to date there are different mutations in this gene including insertional frameshifts in exon 3 and 8, a deletional frameshift in exon 8, and a large 5' and promoter deletion.[31] It has been proposed that as a single active copy gene, the only X-linked FA gene, it may represent a vulnerability point for the genome of cells from obligate heterozygotes. An alternative view is that this protein too will prove to be multifunctional and required for cell survival. Indeed, studies of the methylation status of the gene showed that FANCB inactivation seems to be skewed toward the mutated allele.[31]

It is increasingly evident that the function of Fanconi proteins may be lost during multi-step carcinogenesis[32-34] but it is not clear whether the loss occurs early or late in carcinogenesis. Based on serial studies of cytokine responses of committed hematopoietic progenitor cells in humans with FA,[35] we have proposed that acquired loss of FA gene function cannot be an initiating event (such a cell would lose a competitive advantage) and that other somatic changes must occur first to protect such cells from the apoptotic consequences of FA loss.[32,35,36] Two recent findings have supported this model indirectly. First, apoptotic responses are indeed blunted in marrow cells of FA knockout mice with clonal evolution.[37,38] Second, the observation that in FANCB heterozygotes, X inactivation is skewed in favor of the mutated allele, indicates that the mutant cells are less fit to compete with the non mutant ones during development. A FANCB knockout mouse will be required to determine at which stage of development in heterozygotes the mutant FANCB cells are lost. There are likely other nonDNA damage related functions of the FANCB gene given that the affected males have classic FA phenotypes including bone marrow failure, but no data have been developed yet in support of this expectation.

FANCC

This was the first of the FA genes to be cloned.[13] Ten to fifteen percent of FA cases can be accounted for by mutations of this gene.[39] Although there are a number of heterogeneous

Table 2. Some nonFA FA-binding proteins

FA Protein	NonFA Binding Partner	Functional Relevance
BRCA2	Rad51[77,78]	Experiments demonstrating that FANCD1 mutant cells exhibited aberrant damage-induced Rad51 nuclear focus formation [79] led to identification of BRCA2 as a FA-D1 complementing gene. Mutations of BRCA2 that lead to FA disrupt the Rad51 binding region.[80]
FANCC	STAT1	FANCC facilitates activation of STATs by cytokines[64] and probably promotes survival of hematopoietic cells by doing so.
FANCC	hsp70	FANCC/hsp70 binding suppresses PKR activation[28,29] and thereby promotes survival of hematopoietic and embryonal cells.
FANCC	NADPH cytochrome p450 reductase[130]	Unknown.
FANCC	FAZF[131,132]	Unknown. Possible chromatin remodeling function. The relevance of FAZF is suggested by its consistent expression in primitive hematopoietic cells.[131]
FANCC	GRP94[133]	Unknown. GRP94 has anti-apoptotic activity (93) and FANCC may facilitate that function.
FANCC	cdc2[49]	Unknown but results of Kruyt et al[134] suggest the interaction may be functional
FANCC	GSTP1[54]	Unknown
FANCA	BRG1[27]	Unknown. Possible chromatin remodeling function (BRG1 is a subunit of the chromatin-remodeling SWI/SNF complex).
FANCA	Alpha spectrin and XPF[135]	Unknown.
FANCA	SNX5[136]	Unknown. Possible co-chaperone effect of FANCA in SNX5-dependent receptor trafficking between organelles.[136]
FANCG	CYP2E[137]	Unknown
FANCD2	USP1	USP1 binds to and deubiquitinates FANCD2 and probably modulates the FA pathway in this way.[89]

mutations of this gene, two mutations account for most of the known FANCC mutations; the first in exon 1 (322delG) and the other in exon 4 (c.711 + 4A>T, also until recently termed "IVS4+4A-T" is a single base change in the fourth intronic base that results in deletion of exon 4). The 322delG mutation is hypomorphic for some FANCC functions,[40] likely because of a downstream reinitiation site that gives rise to a truncated protein.[41] The c.711 + 4A>T is unique to patients of Ashkenazi Jewish ancestry in which population the carrier frequency is 1/100.[42,43]

Because it was the first gene cloned more is known about the function of FANCC than any other FA gene. Many of the lessons learned about this protein will likely hold generally for most of the other members of the core complex as well. FANCC is a member of the core complex,[44-46] and binds to FANCE which facilitates nuclear translocation of FANCC.[47,48] At least one nuclear function of this protein is to facilitate the FANCD2/BRCA1 interaction in S phase and in cells exposed to cross-linking agents. Another might be to influence cell cycle control because the FAC protein (but not a mutant protein) coimmunoprecipitates with cyclin-dependent kinase, cdc2.[49] Other FANCC-interacting proteins are listed in Table 2.

FANCC Is Required for Survival of Hematopoietic Cells

In mice, the most consistent FA phenotype is hypogonadism,[50-52] but in humans the single dominant early life-threatening feature of FA phenotype is hematopoietic failure that results from excessive apoptosis in hematopoietic cell populations including myeloid and erythroid progenitors.[10,28,53-63] The FANCC protein sets a high apoptotic threshold in normal cells and apoptotic responses of FA cells exposed to certain extracellular apoptotic cues (interferon gamma, tumor necrosis factor alpha, mip-1α, fas ligand, and dsRNA) are exaggerated in vitro and in vivo.[10,28,29,56,58,60,63-65]

For the nuclear core FA complex to account for the hematopoiesis-specific anti-apoptotic function of FA proteins, it might serve to directly govern the expression of genes that encode intra- or extracellular survival factors specifically for hematopoietic cells. An alternative view, one better supported by experimental evidence, is that the FANC proteins have functions independent of their capacity to form "the nuclear core complex" and that some of the FA proteins might even work entirely on their own (reviewed in ref. 10).

FANCC and STAT Signaling

We determined more than a decade ago that FANCC is required for survival of hematopoietic cells.[66] Our results predicted that the FANCC protein either facilitated survival signals or suppressed apoptotic cues. It turns out that FANCC plays both roles. For example, FANCC is required for optimal activation of STAT molecules and the Jak kinase family member Tyk2, thereby facilitating cell survival and preserving interferon responses,[10,64] Recently it has been found that the disruption of this signaling pathway underlies a subtle T-cell defect in Fancc knockout mice.[67] The hematopoietic support function of CD4 cells is also perturbed (Fagerlie S, manuscript in preparation) emphasizing the multi-factorial nature of marrow failure in FA. That is, not only are myeloid and erythroid progenitor cells hypo-responsive to survival cues, lymphoid cells that support survival of progenitors are defective as well.

FANCC, hsp70, and PKR

FANCC also governs the apoptotic threshold by suppressing pro-apoptotic signals. It suppresses the state of activation of the double stranded RNA dependent protein kinase, PKR, by binding to hsp70 (like a cochaperone) and facilitating the association of PKR and hsp70.[28,29,56] PKR exists in an inactive monomeric ground state in normal cells but is constitutively activated in FA-C cells.[56] As a result of this aberrant state of activation of PKR, exposure of mutant cells to IFN-gamma and TNF-alpha hyper-activates PKR and accounts for earlier observations that FA-C progenitor cells were hypersensitive to IFN-gamma[68] and TNF-alpha.[58] Indeed, PKR activity is now known to be increased in primary bone marrow cells of patients with FA-C, FA-A, and FA-G.[29,65] Interestingly, mutations of FANCC, FANCA and FANCG result in enhanced FANCC/PKR binding, and while it is unclear that this aberrant binding per se results in PKR activation (possibly by facilitating a structural change resulting in ground state PKR dimerization) the results do suggest that nonnative FA complexes can create serious pathophysiological consequences.[65]

FANCC and Oxidative Stress

It has become increasingly clear that the FA proteins play a role in controlling cellular responses to a variety of extracellular challenges and stress; biotic, oxidative, and chemical. Results of an ongoing multi-institutional FA transcriptome consortium support this notion. Results of the study will be broadly shared with the scientific community in the future. There is also good biochemical evidence that FA proteins influence the states of activation of key mediators of cellular stress responses, including GSTP1 and ASK1.

Many investigators have long held that a fundamental defect of FA cells is intolerance to oxidative stress.[69,70] In support of this notion, Buchwald's group recently reported that FANCC enhances the function of GSTP1 in cells exposed to inducers of apoptosis.[54] GSTP1 is an enzyme that detoxifies by-products of redox stress and xenobiotics. While FANCC does not directly interact with GSTP1, its influence on this molecule may play a central role in tolerance of extracellular cues of many kinds. Haneline and her colleagues recently observed ASK1 hyper-activation in H_2O_2-treated Fancc[-/-] cells and used gain- and loss-of-function analyses to confirm that the hypersensitivity of Fancc mutant cells to oxidative stress was mediated, at least in part, through altered redox regulation and ASK1 hyper activation.[71]

FANCC Is Multifunctional

Studies on STAT signaling defects in FA cells have also permitted the development of structure-function studies that prove that FANCC is multifunctional. Specifically, a central, highly conserved domain of FANCC is required for functional interaction with STAT1 and conservative mutations of this domain interfere with STAT signaling functions of FANCC but these mutations have no impact on the capacity of the domain mutant to complement in MMC assays.[40] Another mutant (322delG) was unable to complement in MMC assays but did correct the STAT signaling defect. Interestingly, this mutation occurs in FA patients who have mild disease and mild hematopoietic defects.

Studies on FANCC and the Molecular Basis of Mosaicism

Some patients with FA exhibit mosaicism in hematopoietic cells. These cases are ascertained by observing 2 subpopulations of lymphocytes, one sensitive and one resistant to cross-linking agents. Studies on FANCC structure have revealed mechanisms by which mosaicism occurs in such patients and can be used as a model for mosaicism in other complementation groups. Mosaicism can derive from recombination[72] or compensatory sequence alterations in cis.[73] Two patterns of recombination were described in haplotype analyses;[72] the first was a single intragenic crossover between the maternally and paternally inherited mutations and the second was likely gene conversion. In support of the hematopoietic survival function of FANCC, in the majority of the mosaic patients studied, the blood counts were only minimally suppressed.[72]

In summary, FANCC is a multifunctional protein that protects cells from the genotoxic consequences of cross-linking agent exposure by complexing with other members of the FA core complex to participate in the "linear pathway".[21] It also supports survival of cells in the ground state and cells exposed to a variety of biological cues that induce apoptotic responses. It does this by participating in at least three signaling pathways (STAT, PKR, and ASK signaling) at least in part by functioning very much in the same way a cochaperone would function. We believe that in time these nongenotoxicity functions of FANCC will be matched by like functions of the other FA proteins, some of which have domains (e.g., the TPR motifs in FANCG) that theoretically meet standards for cochaperone functionality.[74-76]

FANCD1 (BRCA2)

Two observations converged to reveal the identity of the FANCD1 gene. First, it was known that BRCA2 binds Rad51,[77,78] and second that FANCD1 mutant cells exhibited aberrant damage-induced Rad51 nuclear focus formation.[79] These observations led to identification of BRCA2 as a FA-D1 complementing gene[17] and the confirmation that FA alleles of BRCA2 disrupt the Rad51 binding region.[80] This is not a common allele and because truly null mutations of BRCA2 are lethal in a murine model,[81] the mutations of BRCA2 that lead to FA are likely hypomorphic. The few FA-D1 patients identified to date have presented with early-onset malignancies of both hematopoietic and nonhematologic types.[82]

Monoubiquitinated FANCD2 seems to promote loading of BRCA2 into multimeric complexes on chromatin by binding to the C terminus of BRCA2.[83] Two separate sites on BRCA2 also interact with FANCG.[84] Using the I-SceI endonuclease to introduce a double-strand break at a specific chromosomal locus, Jasin's group found that BRCA2 mutant cell lines are recombination deficient.[85] Therefore, it is likely that these complexes are required for normal homology-directed DNA repair.

FANCD2

The gene cloned by Markus Grompe's group at Oregon Health and Science University[86] led to the development of the "linear pathway model" for integration of FA protein function. FANCD2 associates with RAD51 and BRCA1 during S phase[87] but given the sheer size and likely complexity of these multimeric complexes, the association of these proteins per se is not sufficient to facilitate DNA repair by homologous recombination. Ubiquitination of FANCD2 requires the core complex but efficient ubiquitination also requires the ATR checkpoint kinase and RPA1.[88] Recently the deubiquitinating enzyme, USP1 was found to bind to FANCD2 (Table 2) and suppress expression of the ubiquitinated form.[89]

There is a good deal of uncertainty about the function of the monoubiquitinated form of FANCD2 and its functional relationship with BRCA1 and BRCA2. For example, there were conflicting reports on the influence of the FA pathway on Rad51 and BRCA2 focus formation in cells exposed to ionizing radiation. Ohashi et al[90] recently utilized BRCA2 and FANCD2 deficient cells and cells treated with siRNAs specifically targeting BRCA2, Rad51, and FANCD2 and developed data suggesting that FANCD2 does not have a direct role in BRCA2 and Rad51 associated homologous recombination repair after DNA damage.

This question still requires further evaluation because (1) survival assays were utilized (2) FA cells are hypersensitive to interferon (3) of the known capacity of some siRNAs to activate interferon responses,[91] and this pitfall was not experimentally ruled out.

FANCD2 and Diagnosis of Fanconi Anemia

Inactivating mutations in all FA genes but BRCA2 lead to failure of accumulation of FANCD2 in damage-induced nuclear foci[21] and FANC alleles of BRCA2 interdict accumulation of Rad51 in such foci.[79] Therefore, although it is currently impractical, screening cells for FA lesions could involve microscopic assessments of damage-induced nuclear foci for FANCD2 and Rad51. FANCD2 immunoblots that distinguish the ubiquitinylated and nonubiquitinylated forms of FANCD2 might also be used to implicate inactivating mutations of any known FA gene except BRCA2.[92] In the context of an unambiguous FA phenotype (by MMC assays in the appropriate clinical setting), if FANCD2 is ubiquitinylated the likely complementation groups would be FA-D1 or FA-J. BRCA2 mutants could be then identified using BRCA2 immunoblots which should reveal only truncated versions of the protein.

FANCE

A rare FA gene, FANCE maps to 6p22-p21[93] and encodes a 536 amino acid protein that is part of the core complex[15,94] but plays a role in transporting cytoplasmic FANCC into the nucleus.[48] Mutations of FANCE include a 355C-T transition in the FANCE gene, leading to a gln119-to-ter (Q119X) nonsense change, a G-to-A change at position -8 in intron 5, resulting in false splicing and insertion of 6 nucleotides from intron 5, including an in-frame stop codon, and a 421C-T transition resulting in an arg141-to-ter (R141X) nonsense change.[15]

FANCF

Discovered by complementation cloning, de Winter et al found that the FANCF gene is intronless and encoded a peptide with homology to the N terminus (RNA binding domain) of the prokaryotic RNA-binding protein ROM.[14] FANCF is largely nuclear and is a member of the core complex. Mutations of FANCF described to date are mostly deletions including a 23 base-pair deletion of nucleotides 230-252, a 47-bp deletion (349-395), a 2 bp deletion (484-485), Other mutations include a 16C-T transition resulting in a gln6-to-ter nonsense mutation, and a 327C-G transversion (yr109-to-ter nonsense mutation).

The protein encoded by this gene may function as a super-scaffold, organizing the formation of multimeric FA complexes. The C-terminus of FANCF interacts directly with FANCG and may facilitate the assembly of other FA proteins into the core complex (or other complexes for that matter).[95] The N-terminus of FANCF seems to stabilize the FANCA/FANCG interaction and is also required for binding of the FANCC/FANCE complex.[95]

FANCG

By functional complementation of the Chinese Hamster ovarian cell line UV40, Liu et al[96] cloned XRCC9 a gene that conferred resistance to both hygromycin and mitomycin C. Later FANCG was shown to be identical to XRCC9[97] which had been localized to 9p13. The putative 622-amino acid nuclear and cytoplasmic protein is a member of the core complex[46,98] and is phosphorylated at serines 7, 385 and 387.[99-101]

Survival signaling functions of FANCG involve suppression (in collaboration with FANCC and FANCA) of the proapoptotic double stranded RNA-dependent protein kinase PKR.[65] In FANCG mutant cells, binding of FANCC and PKR is increased.[65] In keeping with the theme that nonnative interactions of FA proteins with signaling proteins in FA mutant cells contribute to pathogenesis, PKR activity is increased in bone marrow cells of patients with Fanconi anemia with mutations in the FANCC, FANCA, and FANCG genes.

There are numerous FANCG mutations. Most result in protein truncations[102] but the sites of mutation are not clustered. In 9 German FAG patients there was a 313G-T transversion in 8 of 18 (44%) mutated alleles.[102] In 7 Portuguese-Brazilian probands Auerbach et al[103] reported IVS8AS-2A-G. The same team also reported IVS11DS+1G-C in 7 French-Acadian probands, 1794-1803del in 7 European probands, and IVS3+1G>C (five Korean or Japanese probands) and suggest that the Portuguese-Brazilian, French-Acadian, and Korean/Japanese mutations were likely to have been present in a founding member of each of these populations. In black populations of sub-Saharan Africa, the incidence of FA is >1/40,000 and 82% of cases carry the same FANCG mutation (c.637_643 del TACCGCC).[104]

FANCG protein is a member of the core complex, associates with FANCA and FANCF, and dimerizes with FANCA in cells exposed to oxidative stress.[23] FANCG has 6 or 7 (depending on the stringency of the consensus sequence definition) tetratricopeptide repeats,[16] elements that facilitate protein-protein interactions and, interestingly, are domains used by other cochaperones to bind to hsc70[105] and hsp90,[76,106,107] raising the distinct possibility that FANCG, like FANCC may integrate with heat shock responses as a cochaperone.

FANCH

There is no FANCH gene. It was predicted from complementation group analysis carried out on cells later shown to be FANCA mutants.[108]

FANCI and FANCJ

Neither of these two recently identified genes has been cloned to date. That they exist is suggested by somatic cell fusion/complementation analyses and/or genetic data.[12] Using immunoblot analyses for FA core complex formation and FANCD2 mono-ubiquitination, Levitus et al demonstrated that both FA-I and FA-J cell lines formed a core complex, that FA-I cells were not capable of ubiquitinating FANCD2, and that FA-J cells did ubiquitinate FANCD2.[12] This placed the theoretical protein encoded by the mutated gene in FA-J cells "downstream" of the FANCD2 ubiquitination step.

FANCL

This was the first of two FA genes (FANCB being the other) identified using a proteomics approach. Specifically, Meetei et al[30] identified, using mass spectrometry, a 43 kDal Fanconi complex associated protein as PHD finger protein-9 (PHF9). The 373-amino acid protein contains 3 WD40 repeats and a PHD-type zinc finger motif and is clearly a key component of the FA core complex. The protein has ubiquitin ligase activity and may play an important role in the monoubiquitylation of FANCD2.[109] In effect, the other members of the core complex may serve as a scaffold that permits the presentation of FANCL to FANCD2 and possibly to other proteins as well. In fact, taking into account the degree to which FANCD2 is conserved throughout evolution[86] it seems not sufficiently parsimonious that a complex of 7 FA proteins has evolved simply to facilitate one post translational change of FANCD2. Experiments are now underway in our laboratory to identify other substrates that might be ubiquitinated by the FA complex.

The mutation described by Meetei et al[30] was a deletion of exon 11 that removed the part of the WD40 repeat and the entire conserved PHD finger. It arose by homozygous insertion of 177bp at the intron 10/exon 11 splice junction.

FA Protein Complexes

The FA "Nuclear Core Complex"

With the exception of FANCD2 and BRCA2, most of the FA proteins are thought to form a large multi-protein complexes.[21,110-114] Inactivating mutations of FANCA, FANCB, FANCC, FANCE and FANCG proteins reduce assembly, stability, and/or nuclear translocation of the multi-subunit FA protein "core" complex.[46,114]

One function of the core complex has been deduced by nicely-designed studies on isogenic FA mutant cell lines. These studies have clarified an emerging relationship between FANC proteins and some functions of BRCA1, BRCA2 and Rad51. First, as mentioned above, certain BRCA2 (FANCD1) mutations can result in the FA phenotype (FA-D1)[17] and the mutations result in failure of Rad51 to localize in damage-induced nuclear foci.[79] Second, it seems clear that inactivation of any one of the core complex proteins interdicts formation of the complete FA complex, one consequence of which is reduced ubiquitinylation and BRCA1-colocalizing capacity of the nuclear FA protein FANCD2.[21] Therefore, accumulation of BRCA1 and Rad51 in damage-induced nuclear foci is required to protect cells from damage induced by cross-linking agents. Moreover, to accumulate in these foci, BRCA1 requires FANCA, B, C, G, and F dependent monoubiquitination of FANCD2.

What else might the FA complexes do in normal cells? Clearly the complex associates with chromatin in S-phase[44] and while there is no biochemical evidence that this is linked with a repair function, it is an appealing assumption in view of the importance of homologous recombination repair in S phase.[115,116] It is also specifically appealing in light of the linkage between the BRCA1/2 pathways and the FA pathway.

FA proteins, BRCA1, and BRCA2 are known to protect cells from cross-linking agent and oxidation induced genotoxicity.[77,79,85,117-119] Other proteins function in these ways as well, including ATR, Mre11, Tip60, NBS1, Rad51, Rad54, Rev3, Snm1, XRCC2, XRCC3, ERCC1, BLM, and Xpf, although none are associated with the disease Fanconi anemia. However, the precise biochemical functions of the FA complexes are unclear. Based on the current literature, it seems most likely that the FA proteins create scaffolds for assembly and proper folding of enzymes and multimeric complexes and that the client substrates of the FA proteins each function to protect the genome and set thresholds for responses to apoptotic cues. It is widely expected that these proteins are effectors of DNA repair (because of their known function in transcription coupled and homologous recombination repair,[85,117,120]) but biochemical studies have yet to confirm this. Moreover, as a reasonable parallel model, the BRCA1 and BRCA2 proteins exhibit other activities than their role in modulation of genotoxicity. They directly participate in transcriptional control,[121-125] cytoplasmic signal transduction,[126] and regulation of differentiation.[124,127] More work needs to be done to clarify the FA-BRCA1 relationships in functional terms.

Other Complexes

The components of the FA complexes are increasing in number as it becomes clear that there is variability from method-to-method and from one subcellular compartment to another. Formation of complexes is a dynamic process that can be influenced by cell cycle phase, or by chemical or biological cues. Using chromatographic analyses Kupfer's group discovered that the FA "core complex" varies between subcellular compartments. The FA core complex exists in a 500-600 kDal cytoplasmic form, a larger 750 kDal cytoplasmic form seen only in mitosis, a 2 MDal nuclear form, and a 1 MDal form bound to chromatin.[45] Interestingly, monoubiquitinated FANCD2 and BRCA2 also interact in chromatin fractions,[83] but because BRCA2 dependent RAD51 nuclear focus formation can occur independently of FANCD2,[90] the function of the D2/BRCA2 complex may have nothing to do with Rad51 focus formation.

As has been described above, the tendency of FA proteins to form large multimeric complexes has been exploited investigatively to discover new FA proteins. Using a global immunoprecipitation method, Meetei et al[128] identified 3 distinct multiprotein complexes associated with the Bloom's protein, BLM. One of these ("BRAFT") contained topoisomerase III-alpha, replication protein A and the core complex FA proteins. Other members of the complex ultimately proved to be FANCB and FANCL.[30,31]

In summary, most of the FA genes have been cloned now and the elucidation of the FA nuclear complex model by Garcia-Higuera et al[21,46,129] has been extraordinarily helpful in describing a unified vision of how mutations of these disparate proteins can lead to the same aberrant response to MMC. There is also a good deal of evidence that separate functions of the FA proteins account for the molecular pathogenesis of the hematopoietic defects and carcinogenesis but it is less clear whether these functions require participation of the other FA proteins or not. The most coherent functional view of FA proteins is that they act as cochaperones creating multimeric scaffolds that set response thresholds for environmental stress. In view of the emerging evidence that FA proteins affiliate with critically important tumor suppressor genes on the one hand, and participate in survival signaling pathways in hematopoietic cells on the other, studies on the function of these gene products have exciting promise for investigators interested in mammalian development, responses to biotic stress, carcinogenesis, hematopoietic control, and the immune response.

References

1. Fanconi G. Familiare infantile perniziosaartige anaemia (pernizioses blutbild und konstitution). Jahrb Kinderhilkd 1927; 117:257-280.
2. Joenje H, Patel KJ. The emerging genetic and molecular basis of Fanconi anaemia. Nat Rev Genet 2001; 2(6):446-459.
3. Alter BP, Caruso JP, Drachtman RA et al. Fanconi anemia: Myelodysplasia as a predictor of outcome. Cancer Genet Cytogenet 2000; 117(2):125-131.
4. Rosenberg PS, Socie G, Alter BP et al. Risk of head and neck squamous cell cancer and death in transplanted and untransplanted patients with fanconi anemia. Blood 2005; 105(1):67-73.
5. Auerbach AD, Allen RG. Leukemia and preleukemia in Fanconi anemia patients: A review of the literature and report of the International Fanconi Anemia Registry. Cancer Genet Cytogenet 1991; 51:1-12.
6. Alter BP. Cancer in Fanconi anemia, 1927-2001. Cancer 2003; 97(2):425-440.
7. Alter BP. Fanconi's anemia and malignancies. Am J Hematol 1996; 53(2):99-110.
8. Sasaki MS, Tonomura A. A high susceptibility of Fanconi's anemia to chromosome breakage by DNA cross-linking agents. Cancer Res 1973; 33(8):1829-1836.
9. Auerbach AD, Adler B, Chaganti RS. Prenatal and postnatal diagnosis and carrier detection of Fanconi anemia by a cytogenetic method. Pediatrics 1981; 67:128-135.
10. Fagerlie S, Lensch MW, Pang Q et al. The Fanconi anemia group C gene product. Signaling functions in hematopoietic cells. Exp Hematol 2001; 29(12):1371-1381.
11. Bagby GC, Lipton JM, Sloand EM et al. Marrow failure. Hematology Am Soc Hematol Educ Program 2004; 318-336.
12. Levitus M, Rooimans MA, Steltenpool J et al. Heterogeneity in Fanconi anemia: Evidence for 2 new genetic subtypes. Blood 2004; 103(7):2498-2503.
13. Strathdee CA, Gavish H, Shannon WR et al. Cloning of cDNAs for Fanconi's anaemia by functional complementation. Nature 1992; 356:763-767.
14. de Winter JP, Rooimans MA, van Der WL et al. The Fanconi anaemia gene FANCF encodes a novel protein with homology to ROM. Nat Genet 2000; 24(1):15-16.
15. de Winter JP, Leveille F, van Berkel CG et al. Isolation of a cDNA representing the Fanconi anemia complementation group E gene. Am J Hum Genet 2000; 67(5):1306-1308.
16. Blom E, van de Vrugt HJ, Vries Y et al. Multiple TPR motifs characterize the Fanconi anemia FANCG protein. DNA Repair (Amst) 2004; 3(1):77-84.

17. Howlett NG, Taniguchi T, Olson S et al. Biallelic Inactivation of BRCA2 in Fanconi anemia. Science 2002; 297(5581):606-9.
18. Bagby Jr GC. Genetic basis of Fanconi anemia. Curr Opin Hematol 2003; 10(1):68-76.
19. Levran O, Diotti R, Pujara K et al. Spectrum of sequence variations in the FANCA gene: An International Fanconi Anemia Registry (IFAR) study. Hum Mutat 2005; 25(2):142-149.
20. Morgan NV, Tipping AJ, Joenje H et al. High frequency of large intragenic deletions in the Fanconi anemia group A gene. Am J Hum Genet 1999; 65(5):1330-1341.
21. Garcia-Higuera I, Taniguchi T, Ganesan S et al. Interaction of the Fanconi Anemia Proteins and BRCA1 in a Common Pathway. Mol Cell 2001; 7(2):249-262.
22. Folias A, Matkovic M, Bruun D et al. BRCA1 interacts directly with the Fanconi anemia protein FANCA. Hum Mol Genet 2002; 11(21):2591-2597.
23. Park SJ, Ciccone SLM, Beck BD et al. Oxidative stress/damage induces multimerization and interaction of Fanconi anemia proteins. J Biol Chem 2004; 279(29):30053-30059.
24. Yagasaki H, Adachi D, Oda T et al. A cytoplasmic serine protein kinase binds and may regulate the Fanconi anemia protein FANCA. Blood 2001; 98(13):3650-3657.
25. Otsuki T, Nagashima T, Komatsu N et al. Phosphorylation of Fanconi anemia protein, FANCA, is regulated by Akt kinase. Biochem Biophys Res Commun 2002; 291(3):628-634.
26 Otsuki T, Young DB, Sasaki DT et al. Fanconi anemia protein complex is a novel target of the IKK signalsome. J Cell Biochem 2002; 86(4):613-623.
27. Otsuki T, Furukawa Y, Ikeda K et al. Fanconi anemia protein, FANCA, associates with BRG1, a component of the human SWI/SNF complex. Hum Mol Genet 2001; 10(23):2651-2660.
28. Pang Q, Keeble W, Christianson TA et al. FANCC interacts with hsp70 to protect hematopoietic cells from IFNg/TNFa- mediated cytotoxicity. EMBO J 2001; 20(16):4478-4489.
29. Pang QS, Christianson TA, Keeble W et al. The anti-apoptotic function of Hsp70 in the interferon-inducible double-stranded RNA-dependent protein kinase-mediated death signaling pathway requires the Fanconi anemia protein, FANCC. J Biol Chem 2002; 277(51):49638-49643.
30. Meetei AR, de Winter JP, Medhurst AL et al. A novel ubiquitin ligase is deficient in Fanconi anemia. Nat Genet 2003; 35(2):165-170.
31. Meetei AR, Levitus M, Xue Y et al. X-linked inheritance of Fanconi anemia complementation group B. Nat Genet 2004; 36(11):1219-1224.
32. Lensch MW, Tischkowitz M, Christianson TA et al. Acquired FANCA dysfunction and cytogenetic instability in adult acute myelogenous leukemia. Blood 2003; 102(1):7-16.
33. Couch FJ, Johnson MR, Rabe K et al. Germ line Fanconi anemia complementation group C mutations and pancreatic cancer. Cancer Res 2005; 65(2):383-386.
34. Taniguchi T, Tischkowitz M, Ameziane N et al. Disruption of the Fanconi anemia-BRCA pathway in cisplatin-sensitive ovarian tumors. Nat Med 2003; 9(5):568-574.
35. Lensch MW, Rathbun RK, Olson SB et al. Selective pressure as an essential force in molecular evolution of myeloid leukemic clones: A view from the window of Fanconi anemia. Leukemia 1999; 13(11):1784-1789.
36. Bagby GC, Olson SB. Cisplatin and the sensitive cell. Nat Med 2003; 9(5):513-514.
37. Haneline LS, Li X, Ciccone SL et al. Retroviral-mediated expression of recombinant Fancc enhances the repopulating ability of Fancc -/- hematopoietic stem cells and decreases the risk of clonal evolution. Blood 2003; 101(4):1299-307.
38. Li X, Le Beau MM, Ciccone S et al. Ex vivo culture of Fancc -/- stem/ progenitor cells predisposes cells to undergo apoptosis and surviving stem/progenitor cells display cytogenetic abnormalities and an increased risk of malignancy. Blood 2005; 105(9):3465-71.
39. Gibson RA, Morgan NV, Goldstein LH et al. Novel mutations and polymorphisms in the Fanconi anemia group C gene. Hum Mutat 1996; 8(2):140-148.
40. Pang Q, Christianson TA, Keeble W et al. The Fanconi anemia complementation group C gene product: Structural evidence of multifunctionality. Blood 2001; 98(5):1392-1401.
41. Yamashita T, Wu N, Kupfer G et al. Clinical variability of fanconi anemia (type C) results from expression of an amino terminal truncated fanconi anemia complementation group C polypeptide with partial activity. Blood 1996; 87:4424-4432.
42. Whitney MA, Jakobs P, Kaback M et al. The Ashkenazi Jewish Fanconi anemia mutation: Incidence among patients and carrier frequency in the at-risk population. Hum Mutat 1994; 3:339-341.
43. Kutler DI, Auerbach AD. Fanconi anemia in Ashkenazi Jews. Fam Cancer 2004; 3(3-4):241-248.
44. Mi J, Kupfer GM. The fanconi anemia core complex associates with chromatin during s phase. Blood 2005; 105(2):759-66.
45. Thomashevski A, High AA, Drozd M et al. The Fanconi anemia core complex forms 4 different sized complexes in different subcellular compartments. J Biol Chem 2004; 279(25):26201-9.

46. Garcia-Higuera I, Kuang Y, Naf D et al. Fanconi anemia proteins FANCA, FANCC, and FANCG/XRCC9 interact in a functional nuclear complex. Mol Cell Biol 1999; 19(7):4866-4873.
47. Gordon SM, Buchwald M. The Fanconi anemia protein complex: Mapping protein interactions in the yeast two- and three-hybrid systems. Blood 2003; 102(1):136-141.
48. Taniguchi T, D'Andrea AD. The Fanconi anemia protein, FANCE, promotes the nuclear accumulation of FANCC. Blood 2002; 100(7):2457-2462.
49. Kupfer GM, Yamashita T, Naf D et al. The Fanconi anemia polypeptide, FAC, binds to the cyclin- dependent kinase, cdc2. Blood 1997; 90:1047-1054.
50. Nadler JJ, Braun RE. Fanconi anemia complementation group C is required for proliferation of murine primordial germ cells. Genesis 2000; 27(3):117-123.
51. Cheng NC, van de Vrugt HJ, Van der Valk MA et al. Mice with a targeted disruption of the Fanconi anemia homolog Fanca. Hum Mol Genet 2000; 9(12):1805-1811.
52. Koomen M, Cheng NC, van de Vrugt HJ et al. Reduced fertility and hypersensitivity to mitomycin C characterize Fancg/Xrcc9 null mice. Hum Mol Genet 2002; 11(3):273-281.
53. Cumming RC, Liu JM, Youssoufian H et al. Suppression of apoptosis in hematopoietic factor-dependent progenitor cell lines by expression of the FAC gene. Blood 1996; 88(12):4558-4567.
54. Cumming RC, Lightfoot J, Beard K et al. Fanconi anemia group C protein prevents apoptosis in hematopoietic cells through redox regulation of GSTP1. Nat Med 2001; 7(7):814-820.
55. Maciejewski JP, Selleri C, Sato T et al. Increased expression of Fas antigen on bone marrow CD34$^+$ cells of patients with aplastic anaemia. Br J Haematol 1995; 91:245-252.
56. Pang Q, Keeble W, Diaz J et al. Role of double-stranded RNA-dependent protein kinase in mediating hypersensitivity of Fanconi anemia complementation group C cells to interferon gamma, tumor necrosis factor-alpha, and double-stranded RNA. Blood 2001; 97(6):1644-1652.
57. Wang J, Otsuki T, Youssoufian H et al. Overexpression of the Fanconi anemia group C gene (FAC) protects hematopoietic progenitors from death induced by Fas-mediated apoptosis. Cancer Res 1998; 58(16):3538-3541.
58. Otsuki T, Nagakura S, Wang J et al. Tumor necrosis factor-alpha and CD95 ligation suppress erythropoiesis in Fanconi anemia C gene knockout mice. J Cell Physiol 1999; 179(1):79-86.
59. Fagerlie SR, Diaz J, Christianson TA et al. Functional correction of FA-C cells with FANCC suppresses the expression of interferon gamma-inducible genes. Blood 2001; 97(10):3017-3024.
60. Haneline LS, Broxmeyer HE, Cooper S et al. Multiple inhibitory cytokines induce deregulated progenitor growth and apoptosis in hematopoietic cells from FAC -/- mice. Blood 1998; 91:4092-4098.
61. Koh PS, Hughes GC, Faulkner GR et al. The Fanconi anemia group C gene product modulates apoptotic responses to tumor necrosis factor-α and Fas ligand but does not suppress expression of receptors of the tumor necrosis factor receptor superfamily. Exp Hematol 1999; 27(1):1-8.
62. Li Y, Youssoufian H. MxA overexpression reveals a common genetic link in four Fanconi anemia complementation groups. J Clin Invest 1997; 100(11):2873-2880.
63. Rathbun RK, Faulkner GR, Ostroski MH et al. Inactivation of the Fanconi anemia group C (FAC) gene augments interferon-gamma-induced apoptotic responses in hematopoietic cells. Blood 1997; 90:974-985.
64. Pang Q, Fagerlie S, Christianson TA et al. The Fanconi anemia protein FANCC binds to and facilitates the activation of STAT1 by gamma interferon and hematopoietic growth factors. Mol Cell Biol 2000; 20(13):4724-4735.
65. Zhang XL, Li J, Sejas DP et al. The Fanconi anemia proteins functionally interact with the protein kinase regulated by RNA (PKR). J Biol Chem 2004; 279(42):43910-43919.
66. Segal GM, Magenis RE, Brown M et al. Repression of Fanconi anemia gene (FACC) expression inhibits growth of hematopoietic progenitor cells. J Clin Invest 1994; 94(2):846-852.
67. Fagerlie SR, Koretsky T, Torok-Storb B et al. Impaired type I IFN-induced Jak/STAT signaling in FA-C cells and abnormal CD4$^+$ Th cell subsets in Fancc$^{-/-}$ mice. J Immunol 2004; 173(6):3863-3870.
68. Whitney MA, Royle G, Low MJ et al. Germ cell defects and hematopoietic hypersensitivity to g-interferon in mice with a targeted disruption of the Fanconi anemia C gene. Blood 1996; 88:49-58.
69. Pagano G. Mitomycin C and diepoxybutane action mechanisms and FANCC protein functions: Further insights into the role for oxidative stress in Fanconi's anaemia phenotype. Carcinogenesis 2000; 21(5):1067-1068.
70. Clarke AA, Philpott NJ, Gordon-Smith EC et al. The sensitivity of Fanconi anaemia group C cells to apoptosis induced by mitomycin C is due to oxygen radical generation, not DNA crosslinking. Br J Haematol 1997; 96(2):240-247.
71. Saadatzadeh MR, Bijangi-Vishehsaraei K, Hong P et al. Oxidant hypersensitivity of Fanconi anemia type C deficient cells is dependent on a redox-regulated apoptotic pathway. J Biol Chem 2004; 279(16):16805-12.

72. Lo Ten Foe JR, Kwee ML, Rooimans MA et al. Somatic mosaicism in Fanconi anemia: Molecular basis and clinical significance. Eur J Hum Genet 1997; 5:137-148.
73. Waisfisz Q, Morgan NV, Savino M et al. Spontaneous functional correction of homozygous Fanconi anaemia alleles reveals novel mechanistic basis for reverse mosaicism. Nat Genet 1999; 22(4):379-383.
74. Brinker A, Scheufler C, Von Der MF et al. Ligand discrimination by TPR domains. Relevance and selectivity of EEVD-recognition in Hsp70 x Hop x Hsp90 complexes. J Biol Chem 2002; 277(22):19265-19275.
75. Chen S, Sullivan WP, Toft DO et al. Differential interactions of p23 and the TPR-containing proteins Hop, Cyp40, FKBP52 and FKBP51 with Hsp90 mutants. Cell Stress Chaperones 1998; 3(2):118-129.
76. Prodromou C, Siligardi G, O'Brien R et al. Regulation of Hsp90 ATPase activity by tetratricopeptide repeat (TPR)-domain cochaperones. EMBO J 1999; 18(3):754-762.
77. Davies AA, Masson J, McIlwraith MJ et al. Role of BRCA2 in control of the RAD51 recombination and DNA repair protein. Mol Cell 2001; 7(2):273-282.
78. Marmorstein LY, Ouchi T, Aaronson SA. The BRCA2 gene product functionally interacts with p53 and RAD51. Proc Natl Acad Sci USA 1998; 95(23):13869-13874.
79. Godthelp BC, Artwert F, Joenje H et al. Impaired DNA damage-induced nuclear Rad51 foci formation uniquely characterizes Fanconi anemia group D1. Oncogene 2002; 21(32):5002-5005.
80. Stewart G, Elledge SJ. The two faces of BRCA2, a FANCtastic discovery. Mol Cell 2002; 10(1):2-4.
81. Ludwig T, Chapman DL, Papaioannou VE et al. Targeted mutations of breast cancer susceptibility gene homologs in mice: Lethal phenotypes of Brca1, Brca2, Brca1/Brca2, Brca1/p53, and Brca2/p53 nullizygous embryos. Genes Dev 1997; 11(10):1226-1241.
82. Hirsch B, Shimamura A, Moreau L et al. Association of biallelic BRCA2/FANCD1 mutations with spontaneous chromosomal instability and solid tumors of childhood. Blood 2004; 103(7):2554-2559.
83. Wang X, Andreassen PR, D'Andrea AD. Functional interaction of monoubiquitinated FANCD2 and BRCA2/FANCD1 in chromatin. Mol Cell Biol 2004; 24(13):5850-5862.
84. Hussain S, Witt E, Huber PAJ et al. Direct interaction of the Fanconi anaemia protein FANCG with BRCA2/FANCD1. Hum Mol Genet 2003; 12(19):2503-2510.
85. Moynahan ME, Pierce AJ, Jasin M. BRCA2 is required for homology-directed repair of chromosomal breaks. Mol Cell 2001; 7(2):263-272.
86. Timmers C, Taniguchi T, Hejna J et al. Positional cloning of a novel Fanconi anemia gene, FANCD2. Mol Cell 2001; 7(2):241-248.
87. Taniguchi T, Garcia-Higuera I, Andreassen PR et al. S-phase-specific interaction of the Fanconi anemia protein, FANCD2, with BRCA1 and RAD51. Blood 2002; 100(7):2414-2420.
88. Andreassen PR, D'Andrea AD, Taniguchi T. ATR couples FANCD2 monoubiquitination to the DNA-damage response. Genes Dev 2004; 18(16):1958-1963.
89. Nijman SM, Huang TT, Dirac AM et al. The deubiquitinating enzyme USP1 regulates the Fanconi anemia pathway. Mol Cell 2005; 17(3):331-339.
90. Ohashi A, Zdzienicka MZ, Chen J et al. FANCD2 functions independently of BRCA2 and RAD51 associated homologous recombination in response to DNA damage. J Biol Chem 2005; 280(15):14877-83.
91. Sledz CA, Holko M, de Veer MJ et al. Activation of the interferon system by short-interfering RNAs. Nat Cell Biol 2003; 5(9):834-839.
92. Shimamura A, Montes DO, Svenson JL et al. A novel diagnostic screen for defects in the Fanconi anemia pathway. Blood 2002; 100(13):4649-4654.
93. Waisfisz Q, Saar K, Morgan NV et al. The Fanconi anemia group E gene, FANCE, maps to chromosome 6p. Am J Hum Genet 1999; 64(5):1400-1405.
94. Pace P, Johnson M, Tan WM et al. FANCE: The link between Fanconi anaemia complex assembly and activity. EMBO J 2002; 21(13):3414-3423.
95. Léveillé F, Blom E, Medhurst AL et al. The Fanconi anemia gene product FANCF is a flexible adaptor protein. J Biol Chem 2004; 279(38):39421-39430.
96. Liu N, Lamerdin JE, Tucker JD et al. The human XRCC9 gene corrects chromosomal instability and mutagen sensitivities in CHO UV40 cells. Proc Natl Acad Sci USA 1997; 94(17):9232-9237.
97. de Winter JP, Waisfisz Q, Rooimans MA et al. The Fanconi anaemia group G gene FANCG is identical with XRCC9. Nat Genet 1998; 20(3):281-283.
98. Kuang Y, Garcia-Higuera I, Moran A et al. Carboxy terminal region of the Fanconi anemia protein, FANCG/XRCC9, is required for functional activity. Blood 2000; 96(5):1625-1632.
99. Futaki M, Watanabe S, Kajigaya S et al. Fanconi anemia protein, FANCG, is a phosphoprotein and is upregulated with FANCA after TNF-alpha treatment. Biochem Biophys Res Commun 2001; 281(2):347-351.

100. Mi J, Qiao F, Wilson JB et al. FANCG is phosphorylated at serines 383 and 387 during mitosis. Mol Cell Biol 2004; 24(19):8576-8585.
101. Qiao FY, Mi J, Wilson JB et al. Phosphorylation of Fanconi anemia (FA) complementation group G protein, FANCG, at serine 7 is important for function of the FA pathway. J Biol Chem 2004; 279(44):46035-46045.
102. Demuth I, Wlodarski M, Tipping AJ et al. Spectrum of mutations in the Fanconi anaemia group G gene, FANCG/XRCC9. Eur J Hum Genet 2000; 8(11):861-868.
103. Auerbach AD, Greenbaum J, Pujara K et al. Spectrum of sequence variation in the FANCG gene: An International Fanconi Anemia Registry (IFAR) study. Hum Mutat 2003; 21(2):158-168.
104. Morgan NV, Essop F, Demuth I et al. A common Fanconi Anemia mutation in black populations of sub-Saharan Africa. Blood 2005; 105(9):3542-4.
105. Liu FH, Wu SJ, Hu SM et al. Specific interaction of the 70-kDa heat shock cognate protein with the tetratricopeptide repeats. J Biol Chem 1999; 274(48):34425-34432.
106. Russell LC, Whitt SR, Chen MS et al. Identification of conserved residues required for the binding of a tetratricopeptide repeat domain to heat shock protein 90. J Biol Chem 1999; 274(29):20060-20063.
107. Scheufler C, Brinker A, Bourenkov G et al. Structure of TPR domain-peptide complexes: Critical elements in the assembly of the Hsp70-Hsp90 multichaperone machine. Cell 2000; 101(2):199-210.
108. Joenje H, Levitus M, Waisfisz Q et al. Complementation analysis in fanconi anemia: Assignment of the reference FA-H Patient to Group A. Am J Hum Genet 2000; 67(3):759-762.
109. Meetei AR, Yan Z, Wang W. FANCL Replaces BRCA1 as the likely ubiquitin ligase responsible for FANCD2 monoubiquitination. Cell Cycle 2004; 3(2):179-181.
110. de Winter JP, van Der WL, De Groot J et al. The Fanconi anemia protein FANCF forms a nuclear complex with FANCA, FANCC and FANCG. Hum Mol Genet 2000; 9(18):2665-2674.
111. Garcia-Higuera I, Kuang Y, Denham J et al. The Fanconi anemia proteins FANCA and FANCG stabilize each other and promote the nuclear accumulation of the Fanconi anemia complex. Blood 2000; 96(9):3224-3230.
112. Medhurst AL, Huber PA, Waisfisz Q et al. Direct interactions of the five known Fanconi anaemia proteins suggest a common functional pathway. Hum Mol Genet 2001; 10(4):423-429.
113. Waisfisz Q, de Winter JP, Kruyt FA et al. A physical complex of the Fanconi anemia proteins FANCG/XRCC9 and FANCA. Proc Natl Acad Sci USA 1999; 96(18):10320-10325.
114. Kupfer GM, Näf D, Suliman A et al. The Fanconi anaemia proteins, FAA and FAC, interact to form a nuclear complex. Nature Genet 1997; 17:487-490.
115. Hirano S, Yamamoto K, Ishiai M et al. Functional relationships of FANCC to homologous recombination, translesion synthesis, and BLM. EMBO J 2005; 24(2):418-427.
116. Rothfuss A, Grompe M. Repair kinetics of genomic interstrand DNA cross-links: Evidence for DNA double-strand break-dependent activation of the Fanconi anemia/BRCA pathway. Mol Cell Biol 2004; 24(1):123-134.
117. Xia F, Taghian DG, DeFrank JS et al. Deficiency of human BRCA2 leads to impaired homologous recombination but maintains normal nonhomologous end joining. Proc Natl Acad Sci USA 2001; 98(15):8644-8649.
118. Gowen LC, Avrutskaya AV, Latour AM et al. BRCA1 required for transcription-coupled repair of oxidative DNA damage. Science 1998; 281(5379):1009-1012.
119. Husain A, He GS, Venkatraman ES et al. BRCA1 up-regulation is associated with repair-mediated resistance to cis-diamminedichloroplatinum(II). Cancer Res 1998; 58(6):1120-1123.
120. Le Page F, Randrianarison V, Marot D et al. BRCA1 and BRCA2 are necessary for the transcription-coupled repair of the oxidative 8-oxoguanine lesion in human cells. Cancer Res 2000; 60(19):5548-5552.
121. Aprelikova O, Pace AJ, Fang B et al. BRCA1 is a selective coactivator of 14-3-3 sigma gene transcription in mouse embryonic stem cells. J Biol Chem 2001; 276(28):25647-25650.
122. Yarden RI, Brody LC. BRCA1 interacts with components of the histone deacetylase complex. Proc Natl Acad Sci USA 1999; 96(9):4983-4988.
123. Zhang HB, Somasundaram K, Peng Y et al. BRCA1 physically associates with p53 and stimulates its transcriptional activity. Oncogene 1998; 16(13):1713-1721.
124. Zheng L, Li S, Boyer TG et al. Lessons learned from BRCA1 and BRCA2. Oncogene 2000; 19(53):6159-6175.
125. Siddique H, Zou JP, Rao VN et al. The BRCA2 is a histone acetyltransferase. Oncogene 1998; 16(17):2283-2285.
126. Gao B, Shen XN, Kunos G et al. Constitutive activation of JAK-STAT3 signaling by BRCA1 in human prostate cancer cells. FEBS Lett 2001; 488(3):179-184.

127. Kubista M, Rosner M, Kubista E et al. Brca1 regulates in vitro differentiation of mammary epithelial cells. Oncogene 2002; 21(31):4747-4756.
128. Meetei AR, Sechi S, Wallisch M et al. A multiprotein nuclear complex connects Fanconi anemia and Bloom syndrome. Mol Cell Biol 2003; 23(10):3417-3426.
129. Garcia-Higuera I, Kuang Y, D'Andrea AD. The molecular and cellular biology of Fanconi anemia. Curr Opin Hematol 1999; 6(2):83-88.
130. Kruyt FA, Hoshino T, Liu JM et al. Abnormal microsomal detoxification implicated in Fanconi anemia group C by interaction of the FAC protein with NADPH cytochrome P450 reductase. Blood 1998; 92(9):3050-3056.
131. Dai MS, Chevallier N, Stone S et al. The effects of the Fanconi anemia zinc finger (FAZF) on cell cycle, apoptosis, and proliferation are differentiation stage-specific. J Biol Chem 2002; 277(29):26327-26334.
132. Hoatlin ME, Zhi Y, Ball H et al. A novel BTB/POZ transcriptional repressor protein interacts with the fanconi anemia group C protein and PLZF. Blood 1999; 94(11):3737-3747.
133. Hoshino T, Wang JX, Devetten MP et al. Molecular chaperone GRP94 binds to the Fanconi anemia group C protein and regulates its intracellular expression. Blood 1998; 91(11):4379-4386.
134. Kruyt FA, Dijkmans LM, Arwert F et al. Involvement of the Fanconi's anemia protein FAC in a pathway that signals to the cyclin B/cdc2 kinase. Cancer Res 1997; 57(11):2244-2251.
135. Sridharan D, Brown M, Lambert WC et al. Nonerythroid alphaII spectrin is required for recruitment of FANCA and XPF to nuclear foci induced by DNA interstrand cross-links. J Cell Sci 2003; 116(Pt 5):823-835.
136. Otsuki T, Kajigaya S, Ozawa K et al. SNX5, a new member of the sorting nexin family, binds to the Fanconi anemia complementation group A protein. Biochem Biophys Res Commun 1999; 265(3):630-635.
137. Futaki M, Igarashi T, Watanabe S et al. The FANCG Fanconi anemia protein interacts with CYP2E1: Possible role in protection against oxidative DNA damage. Carcinogenesis 2002; 23(1):67-72.

CHAPTER 3

The *FANCA* Gene and Its Products

Laura S. Haneline*

Introduction

Fanconi anemia (FA), type A is the most common FA complementation type with mutations in the *FANCA* gene accounting for approximately 65% of cases.[1,2] The FANCA protein is recognized as an integral component of the multimeric FA protein nuclear complex, which participates in activation of the ubiquitin ligase, FANCL, and results in FANCD2 monoubiquitination.[1,3,4] These observations suggest that FANCA has an important role in maintaining genomic stability through regulation of the downstream FA protein, FANCD2. However, emerging data suggest that FA proteins may have additional cellular functions independent of FA complex formation and post-translational modification of FANCD2.[5-10]

The goal of this chapter is to provide the reader with the most current information pertaining to the *FANCA* gene and its products. We will begin with a brief overview of the cloning of *FANCA*, the identification of *FANCA* sequence variations, and the potential hypermutability of *FANCA* followed by an appraisal of studies conducted to elucidate FANCA protein functions. To conclude, a brief discussion of the potential role of *FANCA* mutations in the development of acquired AML will be reviewed. Integration of experimental data from multiple laboratories, including both clinical and basic studies, has significantly advanced our current understanding of the biologic properties of FANCA. Hopefully, after completing this chapter the reader will gain an appreciation for the complexity of dissecting FANCA protein functions and for the importance of additional genetic, biochemical, and molecular analyses to interrogate FANCA's role in maintaining genomic stability and regulating normal hematopoiesis.

FANCA Gene

Given the overall importance of elucidating the *FA* gene responsible for the most prevalent of all FA complementation groups, a concerted effort by multiple laboratories and FA families was undertaken to clone the *FANCA* gene. Initial linkage studies mapped *FANCA* to chromosome 16q24.3 using microsatellite DNA markers and samples from families with an individual previously shown to be in the FA-A complementation group.[11,12] The *FANCA* cDNA (5.5 kb) was subsequently cloned by two independent collaborative research groups using positional and expression cloning methods.[13,14] The *FANCA* gene is large spanning ~80 kb of genomic DNA and contains 43 exons.[15]

Sequencing the *FANCA* gene from FA-A patient samples has demonstrated significant diversity in the type and location of *FANCA* mutations, including deletions, insertions, missense, nonsense, splicing, and frameshift mutations.[16-20] In addition to disease-associated *FANCA* mutations, numerous *FANCA* polymorphisms have been detected, complicating the verification of whether newly identified *FANCA* sequence variations are actually mutations or

---

*Laura S. Haneline—Department of Pediatrics, Herman B. Wells Center for Pediatric Research, Indianapolis, Indiana, U.S.A. Email: lhanelin@iupui.edu

Molecular Mechanisms of Fanconi Anemia, edited by Shamim I. Ahmad and Sandra H. Kirk. ©2006 Eurekah.com and Springer Science+Business Media.

polymorphisms. These findings emphasize the importance of examining a wide range of normal controls with diverse genetic backgrounds to assess for low frequency polymorphisms as well as testing whether the encoded FANCA protein complements FANCA deficient cells to ensure that the *FANCA* sequence variation is a mutation rather than a polymorphism.

Given the large number of identified *FANCA* mutations and polymorphisms, investigators predict that the *FANCA* gene may be hypermutable. Multiple potential mechanisms have been proposed to account for hypermutability of the *FANCA* gene based on the normal *FANCA* sequence and observed mutations/polymorphisms. Some evidence exists to support slipped-strand mispairing (resulting in microdeletions or insertions), CpG methylation-induced mutations (resulting in single base pair changes), and recombination between related *Alu* sequences (resulting in large deletions) as plausible mechanisms involved in the relatively high number of *FANCA* mutations and polymorphisms.[16-18] In addition, the phenomenon of genetic reversion or somatic mosaicism has been detected in a number of FA-A patients, suggesting that *FANCA* hypermutability may in some instances enhance the survival of FANCA deficient hematopoietic stem cells.

Interestingly, a founder effect for *FANCA* mutations was detected within an Afrikaner population in South Africa.[17] Descendants of this ethnic group have a much higher carrier frequency for *FANCA* mutations, similar to the Ashkenazi Jewish population whose carrier frequency for the *FANCC IVS4+4 A→T* mutation is ~1 in 100. The most common *FANCA* mutation in Afrikaners is a large intragenic deletion with breakpoints being identified between two homologous sequences in introns 11 and 31 of the *FANCA* gene, which are highly homologous to several *Alu* repeat sequences, supporting the idea that *FANCA* may be hypermutable.

However, if the *FANCA* gene is hypermutable, then individuals heterozygous for a *FANCA* mutant allele would, theoretically, be prone to developing cancer and bone marrow failure compared to the general population. Though this is an intruging hypothesis, no direct evidence has established that carriers of a *FANCA* mutant allele are at an increased risk to develop cancer or bone marrow failure. Larger studies are currently underway to address this important question more thoroughly.

FANCA Protein

FANCA has no substantial homology to other known proteins. The encoded amino acid sequence of the human (FANCA) and murine (Fanca) proteins are 66% identical and 81% similar.[21] The FANCA protein has 1455 amino acids (163 kDa) and contains two consensus bipartite nuclear localization signal motifs. Not surprising then is the observation that the majority of FANCA is localized in the nucleus, though FANCA can also be detected in the cytoplasm, albeit at lower levels. Nuclear localization is required for FANCA to correct the hypersensitivity of FANCA deficient cells to bifunctional alkylating agents,[22] likely via FANCA participation in the multimeric FA nuclear protein complex.

FA-A patients, like individuals in other FA complementation types, exhibit a number of congenital anomalies. To understand the role FANCA has in regulating normal embryonic development, *Fanca* expression patterns were examined in the developing mouse embryo.[23] In situ hybridization studies demonstrated *Fanca* transcripts in multiple murine embryonic tissues including bone, kidney, liver, and brain, correlating with anatomic sites frequently exhibiting congenital defects in FA-A patients. In contrast, studies using the same methodology conducted by an independent research group reported relatively ubiquitous *Fancc* expression in the developing mouse embryo,[23,24] suggesting either nonoverlapping functions of Fanca and Fancc or differences in the regulation of tissue-specific expression. However, caution should be taken when comparing these studies because in situ hybridization may not be a sensitive enough tool to detect low expression levels and may not correlate with protein levels.

Fanca protein expression was also evaluated in multiple adult murine tissues.[21] Similarly, these studies found tissue-specific Fanca expression, with a high level of Fanca expression in testis, ovary, thymus, spleen, and lymph nodes, lower, but detectable Fanca expression in mammary gland, kidney, and lung, and very low Fanca expression in heart, liver, and skeletal muscle. These studies also suggest that Fanca and Fancc expression patterns are not entirely overlapping since Fancc protein is ubiquitously expressed,[21,24-26] supporting independent functions and/or regulation of these proteins. Given the similarities between the clinical phenotypes of FA-A and FA-C patients, these observations are intriguing yet remain incompletely understood.

FANCA Function

Several experimental approaches have been utilized to investigate the mechanism by which FANCA maintains genomic integrity to protect humans from bone marrow failure and malignancies including clinical genotype-phenotype studies, FANCA protein-protein interactions, structure-function studies, and murine knock-out studies. Data using each of these approaches have provided insight into FANCA biology. Collectively, the integration of these experimental observations advance our current understanding of FANCA functions, given that each approach has complementary weaknesses and strengths. Below is a summary of these data.

Genotype-Phenotype Correlations in FA-A Patients

It is becoming increasingly apparent that distinct mutations within a single gene do not always result in the same clinical phenotype. Understanding how individual *FANCA* mutations impact a patient's clinical phenotype is important for two major reasons. First, genotype-phenotype data can be used to prospectively guide clinical management of patients with a specific *FANCA* mutation given a predicted clinical outcome. For example, if a particular *FANCA* mutation results in early onset bone marrow failure, clinicians may decide to follow patients with this mutation more frequently, possibly proceeding to bone marrow transplantation earlier. Second, genotype-phenotype data may also provide clues into important functional domains within a protein, which has the potential to significantly advance our knowledge regarding FANCA function. While this type of data is clearly important, it is not a trivial undertaking to conduct these experiments, especially for *FANCA* given the high number of identified mutations, polymorphisms, the size of the gene, and the rarity of the disease.

One large study enrolling 172 FA-A patients examined whether specific mutations in the *FANCA* gene correlated with a worse clinical phenotype.[27] These studies showed that individuals with homozygous *FANCA* mutations resulting in no protein expression (null mutations) had an earlier hematologic onset and death compared to individuals that expressed a mutant FANCA protein, arguing that the mutant protein possesses a residual function that protects hematopoietic stem cells. Thus, prospective identification of *FANCA* null mutations may alter the clinical management of FA-A patients with those mutations. Similar genotype-phenotype correlations have been detected for specific *FANCC* mutations with the *FANCC IVS4+4 A→T* and exon 14 mutations conferring a more severe hematologic phenotype than the *FANCC del322G* mutation.[28]

Two large studies examined how the clinical phenotype of FA-A patients compared to other FA complementation types.[27,28] On the surface the results from these studies seem to directly oppose one another. The first study reported data suggesting that FA-C patients have a milder hematologic disease compared to FA-A and FA-G patients,[27] while a second study showed that FA-C patients have a more severe hematologic phenotype compared to FA-A and FA-G patients.[28-31] The apparent discrepancy of these observations is likely due to mutation differences between the individuals studied as well as from differences in ethnic background of the subjects studied. For example, the first study showing that FA-C patients exhibit a less severe hematologic phenotype is probably because a higher proportion (50%) of individuals had the milder *FANCC del322G* mutation compared to FA-C patients in the second study who displayed the more severe *FANCC IVS4+4 A→T* and exon 14 mutations (65%). Information regarding the frequency of null *FANCA* mutations, which results in a severe hematologic phenotype, was not reported in both studies for comparison. Collectively, these data emphasize the importance of genotype-phenotype studies in addition to direct phenotypic comparisons between FA complementation types to counsel families and guide clinical therapies.

FANCA Protein-Protein Interactions and Structure Function Studies

Since the majority of FA patients exhibit an overall similar clinical phenotype regardless of complementation group, numerous studies have examined whether FANCA interacts directly with other FA proteins in an attempt to define how FA proteins cooperate to protect genome integrity. Data from multiple laboratories confirm that the N-terminus of FANCA directly binds to FANCG, while FANCC, FANCE, and FANCF bind FANCA indirectly or weakly in a multimeric protein complex.[32-37] FANCA-FANCG binding stabilizes these proteins, resulting in an increased half-life for both FANCA and FANCG.[32] In addition, FANCF expression has been shown to further stabilize FANCA-FANCG binding.[35] Interestingly, recent studies suggest that the stoichiometry of FA proteins may not be 1:1 in the multimeric FA protein complex with evidence supporting that FANCA dimers or multimers may form.[34,38]

Structure function studies demonstrate that multiple patient-derived FANCA mutants are also capable of binding FANCG with variable affinities for FANCC and FANCF.[39] This observation is intriguing and suggests that while the FANCA-FANCG interaction is required for genomic stability, disruption of this interaction is not the main reason for loss of FA pathway function in FA-A patients. In contrast, perturbed recruitment of FANCC and FANCF to the mutant FANCA-FANCG complex suggests that dysfunctional assembly of the multimeric FA protein complex has an important role in the pathogenesis of FA.

In addition to examining for FA proteins that interact with FANCA, several investigators have employed strategies to identify novel FANCA binding partners to obtain clues regarding FANCA function(s). Interestingly, though FANCA is primarily localized in the nucleus, emerging data suggest that FANCA interacts with cytoplasmic proteins as well as nuclear proteins,[9,10,32,40-44] leaving the potential that FANCA may have a distinct cytoplasmic function in addition to a nuclear function. Recently, yeast two-hybrid screens showed that FANCA interacts with proteins involved in transcriptional regulation, DNA repair, proteosome control, intracellular signaling pathways, and cellular metabolic regulation.[44] Together these observations are very interesting, however no functional interactions have been demonstrated for any of the identified proteins that bind FANCA. Defining functional connections between FANCA and its binding proteins is the next critical step towards advancing our understanding of FANCA function.

To date, little has been learned regarding the regulation of FANCA expression, protein-protein interactions, and nuclear localization. Multiple *FANCA* transcripts have been identified by Northern blot analysis, suggesting that alternative splicing of the *FANCA* gene may be one mechanism involved in regulation of FANCA expression/function.[15,21] However, further studies are needed to verify this possibility. The only data available to suggest a mechanism that regulates FANCA-protein interactions and nuclear localization involves serine phosphorylation of FANCA.[45,46] Originally, it was noted that FANCA phosphorylation did not occur in FANCB, FANCC, FANCE, FANCF, or FANCG deficient cell lines, which also correlated with the lack of nuclear FANCA accumulation.[46] These data suggest that FANCA phosphorylation is required for FA complex formation and nuclear localization. However, in a more recent study examining several FANCA mutant proteins, FANCA phosphorylation was reported to be independent of FANCA binding to FANCC or FANCG,[39] supporting as yet undefined complex regulatory mechanisms affecting FANCA nuclear trafficking and FA pathway function.

While FANCA phosphorylation is required for normal FANCA function, the precise FANCA phosphorylation site(s) and the kinase(s) responsible for FANCA phosphorylation are unknown. Some evidence supports that FANCA phosphorylation is dependent on a phosphatidylinositol-3 kinase pathway, using the phosphatidylinositol-3 kinase inhibitor wortmannin.[45] However, wortmannin has been shown to inhibit other kinases,[47-50] arguing that additional data be generated to substantiate the notion that FANCA phosphorylation is dependent on a phosphatidylinositol-3 kinase pathway. Though these data are important, further studies are required to clarify the specific kinase inhibited by wortmannin, since several proteins are included in the family of phosphatidylinositol-3 kinases. Future studies to identify the protein kinase that recognizes FANCA as a substrate would clearly advance our understanding of FANCA regulation and function. Hence, this is an active area of research being pursued by multiple laboratories.

Murine Knock-Out Studies

Currently, murine models of human disease are a mainstay for biomedical research with the ultimate goals of elucidating disease pathogenesis, evaluating protein function(s), and preclinical testing of potentially novel treatments. To gain a better understanding of how FANCA protects individuals from bone marrow failure and cancer development, three independent groups generated murine models with a disruption in the *Fanca* gene using standard homologous recombination techniques, though unique sites were deleted within the *Fanca* gene in each of the mouse models. In the first model described (exons 4-7 deleted), no Fanca protein was detected by Western blotting.[51] Interestingly, the second model (exon 37 deleted) had markedly reduced Fanca expression, though a faint signal by Western blotting suggests that a hypomorphic Fanca protein is expressed.[52] In the third model (exons 1-6 deleted), Fanca protein expression was not examined due to the lack of an antibody that recognizes the C-terminus.[53] RNA analysis showed successful deletion of exons 1-6, however transcripts were detected for exons 14-18, suggesting reinitiation of transcription and the potential for expression of a truncated Fanca protein. Given the human genotype-phenotype data described earlier, these molecular differences between *Fanca* murine models may be important in understanding why individual phenotypes between the three mouse models are divergent.

Furthermore, investigators have noted genetic background differences when studying mice with the same *FANCA* mutation. For example, testicular weight of *Fanca* -/- mice was lower in a C57/Bl6 background compared to a Sv129 strain,[52] consistent with a worse germ cell defect. In addition, microophthalmia was only noted in *Fanca* -/- mice in a C57/Bl6 strain,[53] suggesting the existence of a modifier gene between the two murine strains. Collectively, these data may explain, at least in part, why apparent discrepancies occur in the field and emphasize the importance of understanding the molecular defects and the murine genetic strains used when comparing and interpreting data generated from different *Fanca* murine models.

Despite some differences between *Fanca* -/- mice, all models demonstrate reduced fertility due to germ cell defects (female > male), hypersensitivity to MMC, and increased chromosomal aberrations, suggesting that each model will be useful in understanding Fanca function. Additional phenotypes observed in at least one of the *Fanca* murine models were reduced hematopoietic progenitors with age, gamma-irradiation sensitivity, and increased apoptosis with ex vivo culture,[52,54] similar to studies with *Fancc* -/- mice.[55,56] Interestingly, studies characterizing the third model (exons 1-6 deleted) detected additional novel phenotypes including spontaneous tumor formation, microophthalmia, and growth retardation.[53] Future studies using *Fanca* murine models should assist in our understanding of Fanca function and interactions with proteins involved in DNA damage surveillance, DNA repair, cell cycle control, and apoptosis signaling.

Acquired AML and FANCA Defects

The high prevalence of acute myelogenous leukemia in FA patients suggests that an intact FA pathway is required to protect hematopoietic stem/progenitor cells from leukemic transformation. Several lines of evidence now implicate dysregulation of FANCA in the pathogenesis of sporadic or acquired AML. First, 79 AML and 79 control samples were examined for *FANCA* mutations using PCR-SSCP.[57] In the AML, but not the control samples, six different missense point mutations were identified in the *FANCA* gene. Unfortunately, the experimental method used in these studies does not detect large deletions or insertions, and given that a high proportion of *FANCA* mutations are large deletions, the *FANCA* mutation frequency may be underrepresented in these studies. In addition, it is unclear whether these were somatic or germline mutations, an important distinction to determine whether carriers of *FANCA* mutations are at an increased risk to develop leukemia versus potential hypermutability of the *FANCA* gene in the general population. Furthermore, only one of the six identified *FANCA* mutations was previously reported as pathogenic, suggesting that further analyses of these *FANCA* mutations are required to evaluate whether FA pathway function is disrupted and are thus also pathogenic.

Another large, complementary study examined for deletions in the *FANCA* gene in AML samples using quantitative PCR.[58] Of the 101 samples evaluated, 4 *FANCA* heterozygous deletions were identified, 35 times the expected *FANCA* mutation carrier frequency. In addition, *FANCA* transcripts were lower in cells from these patients as measured by RT-PCR, suggesting that sufficient FANCA expression may be required for maintenance of genomic stability. Additional support for this notion is provided by a case report describing an elderly patient with AML and reduced FA protein expression.[59] In this case, leukemic cells were markedly hypersensitive to alkylating agents as compared to nonleukemic cells from the same individual. Upon interrogation of FA protein expression in the leukemic cells, investigators detected reduced nuclear FANCA, FANCG, and monoubiquitinated-FANCD2, supporting a disruption in the FA pathway. Interestingly, overexpression of FANCA, but not FANCC or FANCG, corrected alkylating agent hypersensitivity of the leukemic cells. However, FANCA sequencing detected no mutations, supporting aberrant control of FANCA expression and/or nuclear localization as the underlying etiology for FA pathway dysfunction in this individual. Collectively, these studies support a potential role for FANCA in acquired AML and suggest that carriers of *FANCA* mutations may be at an increased risk for leukemia. However, further studies are warranted to elucidate the role FANCA and other FA proteins have in the development of sporadic AML as well as for other malignancies, especially epithelial carcinomas for which FA patients are predisposed.

References

1. D'Andrea AD, Grompe M. The Fanconi anaemia/BRCA pathway. Nat Rev Cancer 2003; 3:23-34.
2. Joenje H, Patel KJ. The emerging genetic and molecular basis of Fanconi anaemia. Nat Rev Genet 2001; 2(6):446-57.
3. Meetei AR et al. A novel ubiquitin ligase is deficient in Fanconi anemia. Nat Genet 2003; 35(2):165-170.
4. Garcia-Higuera I et al. Interaction of the Fanconi anemia proteins and BRCA1 in a common pathway. Mol Cell 2001; 7(2):249-62.
5. Pang Q et al. The Fanconi anemia complementation group C gene product: Structural evidence of multifunctionality. Blood 2001; 98(5):1392-401.
6. Saadatzadeh MR et al. Oxidant hypersensitivity of Fanconi anemia type C-deficient cells is dependent on a redox-regulated apoptotic pathway. J Biol Chem 2004; 279(16):16805-12.
7. Taniguchi T et al. Convergence of the fanconi anemia and ataxia telangiectasia signaling pathways. Cell 2002; 109(4):459-72.
8. Cumming RC et al. Fanconi anemia group C protein prevents apoptosis in hematopoietic cells through redox regulation of GSTP1. Nat Med 2001; 7(7):814-20.
9. Meetei AR et al. A multiprotein nuclear complex connects Fanconi anemia and Bloom syndrome. Mol Cell Biol 2003; 23(10):3417-26.
10. Folias A et al. BRCA1 interacts directly with the Fanconi anemia protein FANCA. Hum Mol Genet 2002; 11(21):2591-7.
11. Pronk JC et al. Localisation of the Fanconi anaemia complementation group A gene to chromosome 16q24.3. Nat Genet 1995; 11(3):338-40.
12. Gschwend M et al. A locus for fanconi anemia on 16q determined by homozygosity mapping. Am J Hum Genet 1996; 59(2):377-84.
13. Lo Ten Foe JR et al. Expression cloning of a cDNA for the major Fanconi anaemia gene, FAA. Nat Genet 1996; 14(3):320-3.

14. Consortium: T.F.A.B.C., Positional cloning of the Fanconi anaemia group A gene. Nat Genet 1996; 14:324-328.
15. Ianzano L et al. The genomic organization of the fanconi anemia group A (FAA) gene. Genomics 1997; 41(3):309-14.
16. Centra M et al. Fine exon-intron structure of the Fanconi anemia group A (FAA) gene and characterization of two genomic deletions. Genomics 1998; 51(3):463-7.
17. Tipping AJ et al. Molecular and genealogical evidence for a founder effect in Fanconi anemia families of the Afrikaner population of South Africa. Proc Natl Acad Sci USA 2001; 98(10):5734-9.
18. Levran O et al. Sequence variation in the Fanconi anemia gene FAA. Proc Natl Acad Sci USA 1997; 94(24):13051-6.
19. Savino M et al. Spectrum of FANCA mutations in italian fanconi anemia patients: Identification of six novel alleles and phenotypic characterization of the S858R variant. Hum Mutat 2003; 22(4):338-9.
20. Callen E et al. Quantitative PCR analysis reveals a high incidence of large intragenic deletions in the FANCA gene in Spanish Fanconi anemia patients. Cytogenet Genome Res 2004; 104(1-4):341-5.
21. van de Vrugt HJ et al. Cloning and characterization of murine fanconi anemia group A gene: Fanca protein is expressed in lymphoid tissues, testis, and ovary. Mamm Genome 2000; 11(4):326-31.
22. Kruyt FA, Youssoufian H. The Fanconi anemia proteins FAA and FAC function in different cellular compartments to protect against cross-linking agent cytotoxicity. Blood 1998; 92(7):2229-36.
23. Abu-Issa R, Eichele G, Youssoufian H. Expression of the Fanconi anemia group A gene (FANCA) during mouse embryogenesis. Blood 1999; 94(2):818-24.
24. Krasnoshtein F, Buchwald M. Developmental expression of the Fac gene correlates with congenital defects in Fanconi anemia patients. Hum Mol Genet 1996; 5(1):85-93.
25. Strathdee C et al. Cloning of cDNAs for Fanconi's anaemia by functional complementation. Nature 1992; 356:763-767.
26. Wevrick R, Clarke C, Buchwald M. Cloning and analysis of the murine Fanconi anemia group C cDNA. Hum Mol Genet 1993; 2(6):655-662.
27. Faivre L et al. Association of complementation group and mutation type with clinical outcome in fanconi anemia. European Fanconi Anemia Research Group. Blood 2000; 96(13):4064-70.
28. Kutler DI et al. A 20-year perspective on the International Fanconi Anemia Registry (IFAR). Blood 2003; 101(4):1249-56.
29. Waisfisz Q et al. Spontaneous functional correction of homozygous fanconi anaemia alleles reveals novel mechanistic basis for reverse mosaicism. Nat Genet 1999; 22(4):379-83.
30. Gregory Jr JJ et al. Somatic mosaicism in Fanconi anemia: Evidence of genotypic reversion in lymphohematopoietic stem cells. Proc Natl Acad Sci USA 2001; 98(5):2532-7.
31. Gross M et al. Reverse mosaicism in Fanconi anemia: Natural gene therapy via molecular self-correction. Cytogenet Genome Res 2002; 98(2-3):126-35.
32. Garcia-Higuera I et al. The fanconi anemia proteins FANCA and FANCG stabilize each other and promote the nuclear accumulation of the fanconi anemia complex. Blood 2000; 96(9):3224-30.
33. Garcia-Higuera I et al. Fanconi anemia proteins FANCA, FANCC, and FANCG/XRCC9 interact in a functional nuclear complex. Mol Cell Biol 1999; 19(7):4866-73.
34. Gordon SM, Buchwald M. Fanconi anemia protein complex: Mapping protein interactions in the yeast 2- and 3-hybrid systems. Blood 2003; 102(1):136-41.
35. de Winter JP et al. The Fanconi anemia protein FANCF forms a nuclear complex with FANCA, FANCC and FANCG. Hum Mol Genet 2000; 9(18):2665-2674.
36. Waisfisz Q et al. A physical complex of the Fanconi anemia proteins FANCG/XRCC9 and FANCA. Proc Natl Acad Sci USA 1999; 96(18):10320-5.
37. Pace P et al. FANCE: The link between Fanconi anaemia complex assembly and activity. Embo J 2002; 21(13):3414-23.
38. Park SJ et al. Oxidative stress/damage induces multimerization and interaction of fanconi anemia proteins. J Biol Chem 2004.
39. Adachi D et al. Heterogeneous activation of the Fanconi anemia pathway by patient-derived FANCA mutants. Hum Mol Genet 2002; 11(25):3125-34.
40. Otsuki T et al. Fanconi anemia protein complex is a novel target of the IKK signalsome. J Cell Biochem 2002; 86(4):613-23.
41. Otsuki T et al. SNX5, a new member of the sorting nexin family, binds to the Fanconi anemia complementation group A protein. Biochem Biophys Res Commun 1999; 265(3):630-5.
42. Otsuki T et al. Phosphorylation of Fanconi anemia protein, FANCA, is regulated by Akt kinase. Biochem Biophys Res Commun 2002; 291(3):628-34.

43. Otsuki T et al. Fanconi anemia protein, FANCA, associates with BRG1, a component of the human SWI/SNF complex. Hum Mol Genet 2001; 10(23):2651-60.
44. Reuter TY et al. Yeast two-hybrid screens imply involvement of Fanconi anemia proteins in transcription regulation, cell signaling, oxidative metabolism, and cellular transport. Exp Cell Res 2003; 289(2):211-21.
45. Yagasaki H et al. A cytoplasmic serine protein kinase binds and may regulate the Fanconi anemia protein FANCA. Blood 2001; 98(13):3650-7.
46. Yamashita T et al. The fanconi anemia pathway requires FAA phosphorylation and FAA/FAC nuclear accumulation. Proc Natl Acad Sci USA 1998; 95(22):13085-90.
47. Vanhaesebroeck B et al. Synthesis and function of 3-phosphorylated inositol lipids. Annu Rev Biochem 2001; 70:535-602.
48. Stein RC, Waterfield MD. PI3-kinase inhibition: A target for drug development? Mol Med Today 2000; 6(9):347-57.
49. Wymann MP, Pirola L. Structure and function of phosphoinositide 3-kinases. Biochim Biophys Acta 1998; 1436(1-2):127-50.
50. Vanhaesebroeck B, Waterfield MD. Signaling by distinct classes of phosphoinositide 3-kinases. Exp Cell Res 1999; 253(1):239-54.
51. Cheng NC et al. Mice with a targeted disruption of the Fanconi anemia homolog Fanca. Hum Mol Genet 2000; 9(12):1805-11.
52. Noll M et al. Fanconi anemia group A and C double-mutant mice: Functional evidence for a multi-protein Fanconi anemia complex. Exp Hematol 2002; 30(7):679-88.
53. Wong JC et al. Targeted disruption of exons 1 to 6 of the Fanconi Anemia group A gene leads to growth retardation, strain-specific microphthalmia, meiotic defects and primordial germ cell hypoplasia. Hum Mol Genet 2003; 12(16):2063-76.
54. Rio P et al. In vitro phenotypic correction of hematopoietic progenitors from Fanconi anemia group A knockout mice. Blood 2002; 100(6):2032-9.
55. Li X et al. Fanconi Anemia type C-deficient hematopoietic stem/progenitor cells exhibit aberrant cell cycle control. Blood 2003; 102(6):2081-4.
56. Haneline LS et al. Retroviral-mediated expression of recombinant Fancc enhances the repopulating ability of Fancc -/- hematopoietic stem cells and decreases the risk of clonal evolution. Blood 2003; 101(4):1299-307.
57. Condie A et al. Analysis of the Fanconi anaemia complementation group A gene in acute myeloid leukaemia. Leuk Lymphoma 2002; 43(9):1849-53.
58. Tischkowitz MD et al. Deletion and reduced expression of the Fanconi anemia FANCA gene in sporadic acute myeloid leukemia. Leukemia 2004; 18(3):420-5.
59. Lensch MW et al. Acquired FANCA dysfunction and cytogenetic instability in adult acute myelogenous leukemia. Blood 2003; 102(1):7-16.

CHAPTER 4

The *FANCC* Gene and Its Products

Susan M. Gordon* and Manuel Buchwald

Abstract

Fanconi anaemia (FA) is an autosomal recessive disorder characterized by progressive pancytopaenia and predisposition to malignancy, often accompanied by congenital malformations. The cellular phenotype of FA includes increased chromosomal instability and accumulation in the G2 phase of the cell cycle, both of which are exacerbated by the hallmark sensitivity of FA cells to DNA crosslinking agents such as mitomycin C (MMC) and diepoxybutane (DEB). FA is genetically heterogeneous, consisting of at least eleven complementation groups, the genes for eight of which have been cloned. *FANCC* was the first gene causal for FA to be identified, and consequently has been the most intensively studied. Loss of function studies have demonstrated an important role for FANCC in the proliferation of germ cells and haematopoietic stem cells (HPCs). Together with the protein products of at least five other FA genes, FANCC participates in the formation of a nuclear protein complex, the formation of which is required for monoubiquitination of the FANCD2 protein. This cooperative action of the FA proteins fits well with the indistinguishable clinical presentation and universal cellular crosslinker sensitivity of the complementation groups. However, despite its ability to participate in a nuclear protein complex and possible involvement in nuclear activities such as DNA repair and transcriptional regulation, FANCC is unique among the FA proteins in having a predominantly cytoplasmic cellular localization. Investigation of possible cytoplasmic roles for FANCC have revealed it to be a multifunctional protein involved in the suppression of cell death in response to a wide range of stimuli including DNA-crosslinking agents, factor withdrawl, dsRNA, stimulatory cytokines and Fas ligation, as well as a having a possibly interrelated role in maintaining of the redox state of the cell.

Cloning and Characteristics of the *FANCC* Gene

The *FANCC* gene was cloned by using a transfected episomal cDNA expression library to functionally complement the crosslinker sensitivity of the FA-C lymphoblastoid cell line (LCL) HSC536.[1] Three complementing plasmids with inserts sized 4.6, 3.2 and 2.3 kb were obtained, all containing the same predicted open reading frame (ORF) of 1678bp with alternatively processed untranslated regions (UTRs). Assuming use of the first in frame ATG, this ORF encodes a 558 amino acid polypeptide with a Mr of 63kD. The predicted protein sequence has no homology to other proteins, although it is evolutionarily conserved in vertebrates, with homology searches finding significant matches in animals as distant as ray-finned fish.[2] Two different 5' UTRs that converge 77bp upstream of the initiation codon represent alternatively spliced exons designated exon -1 and exon -1a. Three different 3' UTRs

---

*Corresponding Author: Susan Gordon—Program in Genetics and Genomic Biology, Research Institute, Hospital for Sick Children, 555 University Avenue, Toronto, Ontario M5G 1X8, Canada. Email: sgordon@sickkids.ca

Molecular Mechanisms of Fanconi Anemia, edited by Shamim I. Ahmad and Sandra H. Kirk. ©2006 Eurekah.com and Springer Science+Business Media.

corresponding to identical sequences truncated at different points generated the 2.3, 3.2 and 4.6 kb transcripts all of which were present on a Northern blot of lymphocytes with the largest being the most abundant.[1]

The human *FANCC* gene was localized to chromosome 9q22.3 by in situ hybridization[3] and Southern blot analysis suggests that the FANCC gene is at least 40kb.[4] The *FANCC* coding sequence contains 14 exons ranging in size from 53bp to 204bp.[5] Skipping of exon 13 appears to be a relatively common alternative splicing event, seen in a proportion of transcripts in both patients and normal controls, although it has not been established whether this in-frame deletion results in a functional protein.[6]

Further characterization of the 5' end of the human FANCC gene revealed that exon -1 is located 5' to exon -1a, separated by a small intron. There are consensus splice donor sites downstream of both exons, whereas only exon -1 and not -1a has an upstream acceptor splice site, suggesting exon -1 is not spliced onto -1a.[7] The large majority of transcripts in lymphocytes contain exon -1[1] and only transcript containing exon -1 and not exon -1a was detected in CD34+ bone marrow cells, even after exposure to growth factors.[8] The sequences upstream of exons -1 and -1a have no TATA or CAAT boxes, but, as often seen in widely expressed genes, CpG islands are present around the putative transcription start sites. Putative cis-acting binding sites are found between exons -1 and -1a and also upstream of exon -1. The genomic region extending from 1500bp 5' of the putative transcriptional start site of exon -1 through the 3' end of exon -1a is able to drive expression of a luciferase reporter in CaCo2 cells. Further deletion analysis revealed strong positive regulatory ability upstream of exon -1 but also suggested the presence of a negative regulatory element in the intron between exons -1 and -1a or in exon -1a itself.[7]

The human FANCC gene contains two p53 binding sites, one in the promoter region (-1295 to -1266) and a second in exon 14.[9] Although p53 has been shown to bind the consensus in the promoter in vitro, luciferase reporter assays showed deletion of this site made no difference in FANCC promoter activity in cell lines overexpressing wild type p53. Wild-type p53 overexpression in human fibroblast and lymphoblast cell lines is nevertheless able to induce transcription of FANCC, although p53 mutants incapable of DNA binding retain part of this activity, suggesting activation of transcription is not entirely due to p53 binding elements in the FANCC gene.[9]

Mammalian Homologs of FANCC

Three overlapping clones representing murine Fancc were isolated from a mouse liver cDNA library.[10] While two clones contained a putative open reading frame of 558 amino acids, the third contained an additional 99bp inserted at nucleotide 1849, resulting in an in frame insertion of 33 residues that extends the predicted ORF length to 591 amino acids. The position of the insertion corresponds to a splice junction in the human gene, suggesting it is an alternatively spliced exon.[10] The predicted amino acid sequence is 66% identical to human, with 79% similarity allowing for conservative amino acid substitutions. Although this is low in comparison to other DNA repair genes, exogenous expression of either the 558 or 591 residue coding regions in a human FA-C LCL corrects the sensitivity to DEB and MMC.[10] The murine Fancc gene has been assigned to chromosome 13 by interspecific backcross analysis.[11]

Cloning of rat and bovine FANCC homologs[12] has provided further insight into the evolutionary conservation of FANCC. The predicted open reading frames of the rat and bovine cDNA are 1674 and 1701bp respectively, with the extra length of the bovine ORF located primarily at the 3' end. An alignment of ORFs from all four mammalian species revealed a 65% nucleotide identity overall. The mouse and bovine 5' UTRs obtained most resemble human exon -1 as opposed to exon -1a. The 3' UTR is not conserved between species, although all contain multiple polyadenylation signals generating transcripts of different lengths.[12]

Alignment of the predicted polypeptides from all four species revealed only 53% amino acid identity or 67% similarity allowing for conservative substitutions (Fig. 1), although all have a

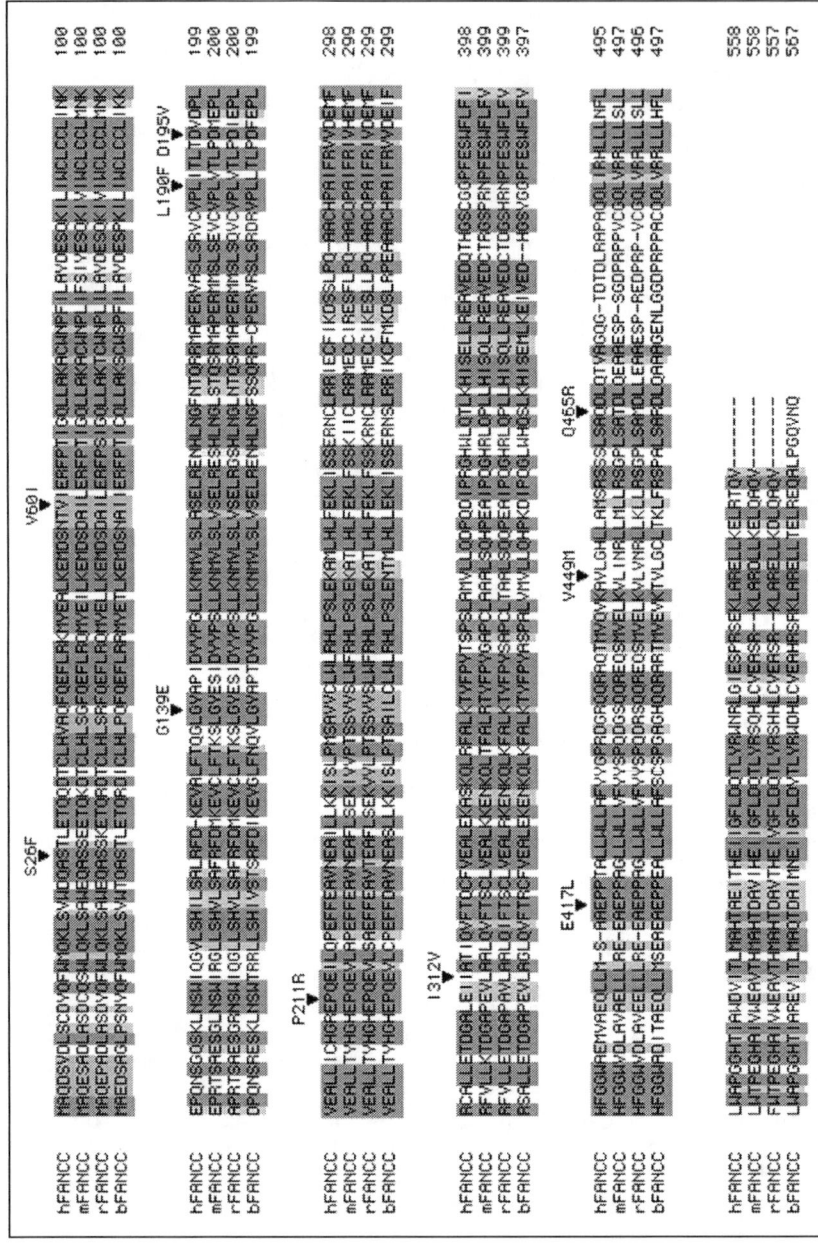

Figure 1. Alignment of the predicted protein products of the human, mouse, rat and bovine *FANCC* genes. Residues identical in all species are indicated by dark shading, with lighter shading indicating similarity if conservative amino acid substitutions are permitted. Human FANCC protein polymorphisms demonstrated not to be causal for FA are indicated above the human FANCC sequence.

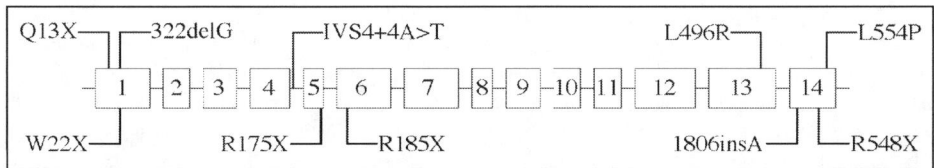

Figure 2. The spectrum of *FANCC* gene mutations observed in patients. Clustering of mutations in exons 1 and 14 is observed. The IVS4 + 4 A>T mutation results in the in-frame skipping of exon 4 or a smaller 40bp deletion likely resulting from the use of a cryptic slice site. Both the R175X and R185X mutations actually result in skipping of exon 6 in some or all transcripts.

similar predicted secondary structure and preponderance of hydrophobic amino acids. Apart from short stretches of 6 to 9 conserved amino acids the degree of similarity is uniform across the sequence.[10] Four putative CK-2 and two putative PKC phosphorylation sites are conserved across species,[12] although an attempt to detect FANCC phosphorylation in multiple cells lines did not generate any evidence that it is a phosphoprotein.[13] The p53 binding consensus in exon 14 of the human sequence is not conserved in the bovine sequence. The bovine *FANCC*cDNA is, however, able to correct the MMC sensitivity of the HSC536 FA-C cell line.[12]

FANCC Gene Mutations

Presence of mutations in the *FANCC* coding region has confirmed its loss of function as the genetic defect in FA-C patients. The HSC536 cell line used in the gene cloning experiments has a maternally inherited L554P missense mutation predicted to disrupt alpha helical secondary structure.[1] *FANCC* transcripts derived from the paternal allele contain a 327bp deletion resulting in removal of exons 1 and 2.[14] Screening of unclassified FA cell lines and patient samples has identified further mutations in *FANCC* for a total of at least ten, with some clustering in exons 1 and 14 (Fig. 2).

Exon 1 mutations include nonsense mutations Q13X[15] and W22X,[16] as well as the deletion of a single G at base 322 (322delG) predicted to generate a truncated peptide of 44 amino acids.[1] The IVS4 + 4 A>T mutation in intron 4[17] generates transcripts with either an in-frame deletion of the entire exon 4 or a smaller 40bp deletion likely resulting from use of a cryptic slice site and causing a frame shift. A nucleotide substitution in exon 5 near the intron 5 boundary is expected to generate a stop codon (R174X), but appears to instead result in exon 6 skipping that maintains the reading frame, with arginine changed to tryptophan.[18] A base pair change resulting in a nonsense mutation in exon 6 (R185X) also results in exon 6 being spliced out of a proportion of transcripts, suggesting this mutation may alter splice site selection.[6] Mutations in the C-terminal part of *FANCC* include L496R in exon 13[16] and the exon 14 mutations R548X,[15] L554P [1] and insertion of adenine at position 1806 (1806insA) expected to generate a frameshift and truncated protein of 526 residues.[19]

Failure to complement MMC sensitivity of the HSC536 FA-C cell line by exogenous expression confirmed the pathogenicity of 1806insA, R548X,[20] L496R[21] and L554P.[22] Remarkably, two siblings homozygous for the L496R (1749T>G) mutation became somatic mosaics when an additional 1748C>T change occurred in vivo at one allele creating a substitution of cysteine instead of an arginine. Complementation analysis demonstrated restoration of FANCC functional activity by this secondary substitution.[21] Overexpression of the L554P mutant several fold in 293 cells has also been shown to induce a level of MMC hypersensitivity similar to that seen in FA cells.[23]

Linkage analysis with three microsatellite markers flanking the *FANCC* gene showed linkage to this locus for 8% of FA families analysed.[24] Large scale screening of FA patients to identify *FANCC* mutations assigned 5.3%[16] to 14.4% [25] of patients to group C, depending on the population used. Seven of the first 100 patients assigned to complementation groups by the European Fanconi Anaemia Research Programme were FA-C.[2]

The two most frequent mutations in *FANCC* are IVS4 + 4 A>T in intron 4 and 322delG in exon1. The 322delG mutation is associated with a mild phenotype, including both fewer somatic abnormalities and later age of aplastic anemia onset compared to all FA patients.[26] Cell lines from patients with 322delG do not express full length FANCC, but do express a 50-kD amino-truncated FANCC polypeptide resulting from reinitiation of translation at methionine 55 (M55). Overexpression of the M55 FANCC cDNA in an FA-C cell line lacking M55 partially corrected the MMC sensitivity phenotype, suggesting the presence of M55 could potentially mediate the FA phenotype in patients with exon 1 mutations upstream of the reinitiation site.[27]

The IVS4 + 4 A T mutation is found in 80% of patients of Ashkenazi Jewish descent,[17] with a carrier frequency greater than 1% in this ethnic group indicating a possible founder effect.[25] In these patients the mutation is associated with a severe phenotype including an earlier age of diagnosis[25] and higher prevalence of several abnormalities including CNS defects.[26] More recently, Japanese patients homozygous for IVS4 + 4 A>T have also been identified.[28] In contrast to Ashkenazi patients with this mutation, no significant difference in severity of clinical phenotype, including age of onset of haematological disease, number of major congenital malformations or development of myelodysplastic syndrome and AML, was seen between IVS4 + 4 A>T homozygotes and other patients. Analysis of surrounding markers did not reveal a founder haplotype in the Japanese patients.[28]

As may be expected given the ability of *FANCC* mammalian homologs with relatively low sequence identity to complement the MMC sensitivity of FA-C cells,[10] the human *FANCC* gene is quite polymorphic. Non-silent alterations causing changes to the coding sequence include G139E,[17] S26F, D195V,[25] L190F, I312V, Q465R, V449M,[16] V60I, E417L[29] and P211R[30] (Fig. 1).

FANCC variants have also been identified in sporadic pancreatic cancers.[31] One clearly inactivating homozygous variant, a somatic 5bp deletion of nt 1903-7 in exon 14 causing a frameshift, has been identified. Another tumour was homozygous for D195V, a variant previously shown to complement the MMC sensitivity of an FA-C LCL. This suggests that this mutation is not causal for FA, but the possibility that it interferes with other aspects FANCC function cannot be ruled out. The functional significance of a heterozygous E521K variant and homozygous M350V variant is unclear, as neither has been previously reported as either a mutation or polymorphism.[31] In another study, a pair of siblings with T-ALL and MDS, one of whom later developed AML, were found to be heterozygous for a 377-378delGA frameshift mutation in exon 4.[32]

Expression of the FANCC Gene Products

mRNA Expression

Human *FANCC*[1] and murine *Fancc*[10] transcripts are detected by RT-PCR in a wide variety of tissues, indicative of ubiquitous expression. RNA in situ hybridization in adult mouse tissues reveals a uniform pattern of expression in all cells,[10] whereas during mouse embryogenesis there is an overall pattern of strong expression in proliferating and differentiating cells that diminishes as cells terminally differentiate.[33] Expression is first detected in the mesenchyme that gives rise to skeletal tissues at embryonic day 8 (E8). *Fancc* is also expressed in non-skeletal mesenchyme including the gut, lung, kidney and site of whisker follicles. Mesenchymal expression generally becomes less abundant as embryogenesis progresses. During the development of bone by endochondral ossification (E13 to E19.5) *Fancc* expression is detected in the actively dividing and differentiating cells of the inner perichondrium, the osteoprogenitors of the inner periosteal layer and in the zone of endochondral ossification, which contains cells derived from both osteogenic and hematopoietic lineages. No *Fancc* expression was detected in relatively mature and differentiated cells such as chondrocytes or osteocytes. *Fancc* expression in the perichondrium of developing digits of the forelimb and in cranial and facial bones formed by intramembranous ossification, is consistent with skeletal abnormalities seen in FA.[33]

In analysis of single-cell murine haematopoietic precursors, *Fancc* is expressed strongly, although at low frequency, in pluripotential precursors and weakly in samples from growing, terminally differentiating populations of monocytes and lymphocytes.[34] RT-PCR to assess mRNA levels in sorted murine haematopoietic stem cell fractions also revealed high *Fancc* expression in lineage-depleted CD34+ cells as opposed to low expression in CD34- cells, suggesting a role at this stage of differentiation.[35] Human *FANCC* mRNA expression in haematopoietic cells is also highest in CD34+ cells from bone marrow, although levels do not change as committed progenitors differentiate in vitro upon exposure to growth factors.[8]

FANCC Protein Expression and Stability

As seen with mRNA expression, exposure to varying levels of TGF-β, IFN-γ, MMC, heat, gamma-irradiation or hydrogen peroxide does not alter FANCC protein levels in LCLs.[8] This is perhaps not surprising given that sensitivity to ICL-inducers is corrected completely by low levels of FANCC protein expression, with greater levels of expression not increasing resistance.[36] FANCC protein levels also do not change in response to hypoxia mimicking agents in a hypoxia responsive cell line.[37] The half-life of wild type FANCC protein in transiently transfected COS cells is approximately 45 minutes, a relatively rapid turnover during which no change in cellular localization and protein interactions are observed with or without MMC treatment.[23]

In synchronized cells, whereas levels of exogenous and endogenous FANCC mRNA expression[38,39] are constant throughout the cell cycle, expression of exogenous FANCC protein is lowest at G1/S, increases during S-phase, is maximal at G2/M, and declines during mitosis.[38,39] Regulated expression of exogenously expressed FANCC requires only the coding sequence and not the 5' or 3' UTR. Inhibitors of the 26S proteasome prevent the reduction in expression at G1/S, indicating this regulation of FANCC expression is dependent on proteasome function.[38]

The discovery of ubiquitinated FANCC also suggests a role for the proteasome in regulation of FANCC. Treatment of normal LCLs with proteasome inhibitors results in cytoplasmic accumulation of an ubiquitinated C-terminal proteolytic fragment of FANCC (p47) that correlates temporally with apoptotic induction.[40] Caspase inhibitors prevent accumulation of p47 as does mutagenesis of putative caspase-8 cleavage sites. Mutation of cleavage sites does not affect the ability of FANCC to restore FANCD2 monoubiquitination and correct MMC sensitivity, and actually enhances the ability of FANCC to delay the onset of apoptosis in response to etoposide. In contrast, exogenous expression of p47 increases sensitivity of LCLs to apoptosis, suggesting that cleavage eliminates the ability of FANCC to suppress apoptosis or that p47 itself is proapoptotic.[40]

Intracellular level of FANCC may also be regulated via its interaction with GRP94, a stress-inducible molecular chaperone.[41] Reduction of GRP94 expression in the rat NRL cell line significantly reduces FANCC protein levels, and induces development of MMC sensitivity in this relatively resistant cell line. Part of the central domain of FANCC that binds GRP94 is spliced out of the IVS-4 + 4 A>T mutant, eliminating the interaction.[41]

FANCC Subcellular Localization

FANCC contains no recognizable nuclear localization sequences and early studies revealed predominantly cytoplasmic localization of the protein in several cell lines,[42-44] with some reports of a smaller amount associated with internal membranes.[42,44] Additional refinement in more recent studies has demonstrated that approximately 10% of endogenous FANCC in LCLs is reproducibly found in the nuclear fractions.[45] Immunofluorescent analysis of exogenously expressed FANCC is highly variable, ranging from predominantly cytoplasmic to predominantly nuclear.[38,45,46] However, FANCC is consistently excluded from nucleoli.[47] Exclusively cytoplasmic localization of the FANCC-L554P mutant[45,46] suggests nuclear localization is not an artifact of overexpression.

In an asynchronous population, FANCC nuclear foci were observed in approximately 25% of cells.[38,47] The exogenously expressed FANCC also colocalizes with endogenous FANCE in nuclear foci.[48] Exogenous expression of FANCE, which contains a putative nuclear localization signal[49] and binds directly to FANCC,[50,51] results in dramatic nuclear accumulation of wild type FANCC but not FANCC containing disease-associated mutations that prevent interaction with FANCE. It is not clear whether this promotion of FANCC nuclear accumulation involves nuclear import or retention.[48] Exclusion of endogenous FANCC from the cytoplasm[13] and overall lower level of FANCC expression in FA-E cell lines is also corrected by reintroduction of FANCE.[52]

FANCC is involved with other FA proteins in a protein complex, the formation of which is required for the monoubiquitination of FANCD2 and correction of MMC sensitivity.[53] Most studies have focused primarily on a nuclear form of the complex containing FANCA, FANCC, FANCE, FANCF, FANCG and FANCL.[13,48,54-57] Recent work has demonstrated that this FA protein complex has at least four forms, all of which contain at least FANCA, FANCC, FANCF and FANCG. There are two cytoplasmic forms sized 500-600kD and 750kD, the larger of which is only present during mitosis, as well as 1MD and 2MD nuclear forms, the smaller of which is chromatin-associated.[58] FANCE is notably absent from the cytoplasmic complexes.[58] The presence of FANCC in cytoplasmic FA protein complexes is not surprising, as FANCC force-targeted to the nucleus is not able to correct crosslinker-induced cytotoxicity, demonstrating that the role of FANCC in mediating this response requires cytoplasmic localization at some point.[36]

Other investigations of FANCC subnuclear localization have revealed its presence in the chromatin and nuclear matrix together with at least FANCA and FANCG. The amounts present in this compartment increase in response to MMC with a time course that suggests cells must first encounter crosslinks during S-phase.[59] Synchronized cells show little change in FA protein content in chromatin and nuclear matrix fractions during G1, S or G2 phase but FANCC and the other FA proteins are not detected at mitosis, implying they are absent from condensed chromosomes.[59] This finding, together with discovery of a distinct mitotic FA complex in the cytoplasm,[58] is consistent with an earlier study of exogenously expressed FANCC in HeLa cells that suggested cells with strong cytoplasmic localization were undergoing or had just completed mitosis,[46] although another study found cell cycle position could not account for FANCC subcellular localization.[38] FANCC from HeLa cell chromatin-associated protein extracts, together with nonerythroid alpha spectrin (αSPIIΣ*), FANCA and FANCG, complexes with a DNA substrate containing interstrand crosslinks generated by psoralen + UVA. It is not clear whether FANCC and the other FA proteins are able to bind directly to the DNA substrate or whether alpha spectrin acts as a scaffold to mediate the interaction.[60]

FANCC has also been shown to directly bind to and partially colocalize in nuclear foci with at least one protein of demonstrable nuclear function, the transcriptional repressor FAZF.[47] FAZF is homologous to and can heterodimerize with the promyelocytic leukemia zinc finger (PLZF), known to play a role in limb patterning via chromatin remodelling.[61] The fact that FAZF protein in CD34+ haematopoietic progenitor cells is highly expressed during early differentiation, declining as myeloid and erythroid cells terminally differentiate, is also intriguing given the phenotype of haematopoietic failure caused by the absence of its interacting partner FANCC.[62]

FANCC in the Cellular Response to ICL Inducers

Cell Cycle Abnormalities

Treatment of FA-C LCLs with low dose MMC causes protracted G2/M arrest mediated by persistent inactivation of the cyclin B1/cdc2 kinase complex preceding or accompanying the induction of apoptosis. In corrected cells, G2/M arrest and inactivation of the cyclin B/cdc2 complex is transient, after which cells resume cycling.[63] Despite a report that FANCC associates with cdc2 in HeLa cell lysates,[39] in uncorrected FA-C cells caffeine-dependent activation of cdc2 releases the G2/M block but does not prevent apoptosis. Thus while the FANCC protein may influence the cdc2 kinase complex to allow G2 to M progression after low-dose MMC, the apoptotic response to low-dose MMC is not directly caused by inhibition of cdc2 kinase activation. At high doses of MMC both FA-C and wild type cells undergo S-phase arrest and high levels of apoptosis.[63]

When exposed to equitoxic amounts of MMC, a similar degree and rate of G2/M arrest is observed in FA-C LCLs compared with corrected isogenic or normal LCLs. This implies that that G2/M arrest in FA-C cells is not an abnormal response at this point in the cell cycle, but a normal response to excessive DNA damage following low-dose crosslinkers.[64] However, while normal and corrected FA-C cells had increased percent of cells in S phase with a discrete peak in late S, uncorrected FA-C cells had a decrease in the proportion of cells in S phase.[64]

Further evidence of an S-phase defect is observed using bivariate DNA distribution methods to analyze the response of LCLs to psoralen plus UVA.[65] Two populations of S-phase cells can be distinguished, replicating and arrested. Normal and corrected FA-C cells are arrested 24 hours after treatment but in FA-C cells replication is continued in S-phase at 24 and even 48 hours. This suggests G2 accumulation is a normal response to excessive damage that reaches that compartment after failure to arrest replication in S-phase.[65] Furthermore, in FA-C as in normal cells, passage through S-phase is required for cell cycle arrest and chromosomal abnormalities in response to crosslinking agents.[66]

Apoptosis

Comparison of the cellular proliferation and viability of FA-C and isogenic LCLs expressing *FANCC* cDNA upon exposure to a wide spectrum of DNA-damaging agents demonstrated that increased cytotoxicity of FA-C cells is limited to cross linking agents such as MMC, cisplatin and nitrogen mustard, whereas other agents including potent free radical producers and non-crosslinking analogs of nitrogen mustard only capable of forming monoadducts did not elicit a differential response.[67,68]

In response to low dose MMC treatment, FA-C LCLs show increased induction of p53 expression accompanied by higher levels of apoptosis compared with isogenic corrected cell lines,[67,69] whereas at higher MMC concentrations similar levels of p53 induction and apoptosis are observed. Despite the observed p53 induction, overexpression of a dominant negative p53 mutant did not increase cell survival, suggesting that p53 is not crucial for MMC-dependent apoptosis in immortalized LCLs,[69] although this appears to differ from the situation in vivo, as discussed later.[70]

It is important to note that not all studies of the response of FA-C LCLs to MMC have agreed that apoptosis is the primary cause of MMC-induced cell death. One study found that at equimolar high doses of MMC, FA-C and normal cells undergo apoptosis at a similar rate, but at equitoxic doses of MMC the level of apoptosis in FA-C LCLs was similar to or slightly less than in normal controls.[71] Further studies using isogenic cell lines failed to detect some of the classical features of apoptosis such as apoptotic body formation, DNA fragmentation and PARP cleavage[72,73] in LCLs following MMC treatment, suggesting toxicity may be mediated by a necrosis-like pathway of programmed cell death.

FANCC Loss of Function

Use of an antisense oligodeoxynucleotide to repress *FANCC* gene expression increased MMC-induced chromosomal breakage in normal lymphocytes and inhibited clonal growth of haematopoietic progenitor cells (HPCs) in a dose dependent manner. No growth-inhibitory effect was observed in fibroblasts or endothelial cells. As the *FANCC* repression did not affect growth factor expression in bone marrow cells, the function of *FANCC* in regulating proliferation of HPCs is likely direct.[74]

Further loss of function studies have been facilitated by the generation of two *Fancc*-deficient mouse models by use of gene targeting to replace either exon 8[75] or exon 9[76] of *Fancc* with a neo cassette. Homozygous null (*Fancc-/-*) mice are viable, with no malformations and no haematological failure or development of malignancy in the first year. Primary cultures of splenic cells and skin fibroblasts from -/- mice show an increase in spontaneous and DEB- and MMC- induced chromosomal aberrations.[75,76] Immortalized fibroblastoid cell lines developed from *Fancc-/-* mice also show significant hypersensitivity to MMC relative to *Fancc+/-* and *Fancc+/+* as shown by reduced cell viability, induction of chromosomal abnormalities, and G2 accumulation.[77,78]

Fancc Loss of Function and Germ Cell Development

Fancc-/- mice, particularly females, have reduced fertility.[75,76] The small ovaries of females have deficient germinal stroma with very few developing follicles. Male mice have testicular atrophy and a mosaic pattern of seminiferous tubules with normal spermatogenesis and abnormal tubules with only Sertoli cells. Both male and female abnormalities are seen in newborns, suggesting germ cell loss is a developmental defect.[76]

Fancc expression is detected by RT-PCR in murine genital ridges throughout gonadal development in both sexes.[79] Comparison of both male and female germ cell numbers during embryonic development revealed a dramatic reduction at all stages examined in the *Fancc-/-* mice relative to *Fancc+/-*. No defect in the migration of germ cells was observed, though a 35% reduction in mitotic index of *Fancc-/-* PGCs at E12.5 compared to *Fancc+/-* reveals a proliferative defect. An additional germ cell survival defect is suggested by the continued decrease in female *Fancc-/-* germ cell numbers after proliferation has ceased.[79]

Fancc Loss of Function and Haematopoiesis

Cultured bone marrow cells from *Fancc-/-* mice have similar erythroid and myeloid colony growth at 2 and 4 months, but a significant reduction at 6 and 11 months compared with heterozygotes.[76] Hypersensitive reduction in progenitor growth in vitro in response to IFN-γ[76] TNFα or MIP-1α (macrophage inflammatory protein-1α) [80] was not age dependent, suggesting cytokine sensitivity could be causal in the progressive depletion of growth potential. *Fancc* is required for prevention of apoptosis in response to cytokines in immature myeloid haematopoeitic cells. Despite elevated apoptotic response, no difference in absolute number of splenic or bone marrow progenitors per organ was observed. Increased suicide in multipotential and lineage specific progenitors implies that a higher proportion of progenitors are cycling in vivo to compensate for the increased apoptosis.[80]

Fancc loss of function is also associated with loss of haematopoietic stem cell repopulating ability in vivo, [81] with long term reconstitution and secondary repopulating ability particularly affected. [82] This is suggestive of a defect in stem cell development potential, an idea also supported by lower differentiation potential of *Fancc-/-* HPCs measured in a single cell culture system. [83] A possible link to the enhanced Fas receptor (CD95) expression in CD34+ *Fancc-/-* HPCs in response to IFN-γ[84] has been suggested.[82] Despite lower overall engraftment, contribution of the *Fancc-/-* cells to lymphoid and myeloid lineages is similar, also indicative of a defect in the pluripotential stem cells.[81] Retroviral-mediated gene transfer of *Fancc* to *Fancc-/-* HPCs enhances repopulating ability.[85]

Haematopoietic progenitor colony assay of bone marrow cells treated with MMC in vitro revealed a marked reduction of erythroid and myeloid colony growth.[78] The effect of MMC in vivo was studied by administration of MMC to *Fancc-/-* mice.[86] Chronic exposure to nonlethal doses of MMC results in a progressive pancytopaenia resulting from a reduction in the number of early and committed progenitor cells not seen in *Fancc+/+*.[86] MMC treatment of bone marrow cells results in a dramatic reduction in number of CD34+ cells but only a slight decrease in CD34- cells, although it is not clear whether the CD34+ population is more susceptible to cell death or whether there is a defect in differentiation from CD34- to CD34+ after MMC treatment.[82] MMC sensitivity of bone marrow cells from *Fancc-/-* mice transduced with retrovirus carrying human *FANCC* cDNA and transplanted to marrow ablated recipients is phenotypically corrected in vivo as assessed by peripheral blood counts following MMC dosing.[87]

As p53 behaviour may be altered by the EBV-immortalization of LCLs, p53 requirement for apoptosis in FA-C cells has been tested in vivo by generation of mice deficient for both genes.[70]

The TNFα sensitivity and apoptosis seen in *Fancc-/-* haematopoietic progenitor cells and MEFs is completely eliminated in double *Trp53-/- Fancc-/-* knockouts, suggesting it is p53 dependent. Low-dose MMC-induced reduction of progenitors is also p53 dependent, although rescue was not maintained at high doses, suggesting a role for a p53 independent pathway. Absence of the *Fancc* gene also significantly reduced the latency of tumour formation in both p53 null and heterozygote mice. In addition, some tumour types not observed in *Trp53+/-* or *Trp53-/-* mice were seen in the double mutants, including malignancies observed in FA patients.[70]

FANCC and Cytokine Signalling

Retroviral mediated overexpression of FANCC in factor-dependent human and murine haematopoeitic progenitor cell (HPC) lines suppresses the onset of apoptosis following IL-3 withdrawal, leading to the suggestion that FANCC may suppress apoptosis in response to normal fluctuations of cytokine levels in the bone marrow microenvironment.[88]

Similarly, HPCs from transgenic mice overexpressing human FANCC were protected in vitro against Fas-mediated cell death induced by either a combination of IFN-γ and TNFα, known to upregulate Fas receptor (CD95) expression, or by a Fas-agonist antibody.[89] Conversely, treatment of *Fancc-/-* murine HPCs with TNFα and Fas-agonist antibody inhibits colony formation in vitro compared to *Fancc+/-*, with BFU-E reduced by TNFα alone.[84] Fas receptor (CD95) expression in the CD34+ fraction of untreated *Fancc-/-* bone marrow is similar to wild type, but its induction in response to TNFα is elevated, with a corresponding increase in apoptotic induction. The effect of TNFα in vivo is similar, with *Fancc-/-* mice transgenic for overexpression of TNFα having increased CD95 in CD34+ cells and spontaneous reduction in BFU-E.[84]

HPCs from an FA-C patient and *Fancc-/-* mice are hypersensitive to the mitotic inhibitory effects of IFN-γ, and IFN-γ-induced priming of the Fas pathway occurs at lower doses of IFN-γ. Colony growth of CD34+ bone marrow cells from an FA-C patient and *Fancc-/-* mice is suppressed by a Fas-agonist antibody whereas Fas blocking antibody abrogates the inhibitory effect of low dose IFN-γ on *Fancc-/-* CD34+ cells.[90] No increased expression of IFN receptor–α or members of the TNF receptor superfamily is observed in patient-derived lymphoblasts or bone marrow cells of *Fancc-/-* mice, either constitutively or in response to IFN-γ treatment, suggesting FANCC suppresses apoptosis via an intracellular mechanism.[91]

The in vitro growth suppressive effects of IFN-γ and Fas-agonist antibodies in both murine and human FA-C bone marrow cells are blocked by caspase-3 inhibitors. In FA-C lymphoblasts, inhibitors of caspase-8 are able to suppress caspase-3 activation, suggesting that FANCC functions upstream of caspase-3 in suppression of IFN-γ-induced apoptotic pathway.[92] However there is disagreement as to whether the level of Fas-mediated cell death in FA-C LCLs is actually elevated [71,73] and the high constitutive level of Fas expression in these cells has been proposed to interfere with the response to Fas-priming.[93]

STAT1 activation in response to IFN-γ is suppressed in the FA-C cell line HSC536, and STAT1 induction is corrected by reintroduction of FANCC.[90] In response to IFN-γ FANCC is required for trafficking of STAT1 to the IFN-γ receptor complex at which point it becomes activated. As STAT1 activation requires FANCC, STAT1 signaling is suppressed in FA-C cells and therefore the excessive apoptosis is STAT1-independent.[94] Despite lack of proper STAT1 activation, protein levels of IFN-γ-inducible genes known to influence haematopoietic cell survival including IFN regulatory factor-1 (IRF-1), IFN-γ stimulated gene factor 3 gamma subunit (ISGF3γ), and the cyclin-dependent kinase inhibitor p21^{waf1} are all constitutively expressed at high levels in FA-C LCLs, bone marrow cells and MEFs. Forced expression of the negative transacting regulator ICSCP (IFN-γ-inducible factor IFN consensus sequence binding protein) in FA-C LCLs does not downregulate the expression of IFN-γ-inducible genes, so FANCC modulates these genes independently of both the STAT1 pathway and ICSBP.[95]

Not all FANCC mutations affect STAT1 activation. The PD4 FA-C cell line, which is heterozygous for the 322delG mutation and therefore contains a mutant form of FANCC protein initiated at methionine 55 (M55), has normal STAT1 activation. Exogenous expression of M55 restores the STAT-1 signaling pathway (STAT-1 DNA binding) in the completely defective HSC536 cell line. This suggests that structural elements of the FANCC protein required for cytokine signalling are, at least in part, different than those required for mediating resistance to DNA cross-linking agents, and may also contribute to the milder phenotype seen in patients with the 322delG mutation.[96] Conversely, alanine mutagenesis within motifs highly conserved in known mammalian FANCC sequences identified mutants able to correct crosslinker sensitivity and restore FANCD2 monoubiquitination but unable to return STAT1 phosphorylation to normal levels in the deficient HSC536 cell line. Lack of STAT1 phosphorylation by these S249A and E251A mutants correlated with reduced FANCC STAT1 interaction, markedly less STAT1 trafficked to the IFN-γ receptor, and increased apoptosis induced by IFN-γ and TNF-γ.[96]

The RNA-dependent protein kinase (PKR), an IFN-γ- and TNFα-inducible protein that influences Fas activity and activates caspases-3 and -8, is constitutively phosphorylated and displays increased dsRNA binding activity in FA-C LCLs and embryonic fibroblasts from *Fancc-/-* mice (MEFs) upon exposure to IFN-γ or dsRNA. Overexpression of wild-type PKR sensitized *Fancc-/-* MEFs to caspase-3 activation whereas inhibition of PKR activity by a dominant-negative PKR mutant reduced IFN-γ and dsRNA hypersensitivity to a greater extent in *Fancc-/-* than *Fancc+/+* MEFs.[97] Modulation of PKR activation in *Fancc-/-* cells is mediated by interaction of FANCC with Hsp70, a protein previously shown to suppress PKR activity and caspase-3 activation.[98] Hsp70, FANCC and PKR have been shown to form a ternary complex in LCLs.[99] Mutants of FANCC blocking interaction with Hsp70 fail to inhibit PKR kinase activity and do not give protection from IFN-γ /TNFα induced cytotoxicity. Repression of HSP70 expression in normal lymphoblasts causes greater susceptibility to IFN-γ and TNFα, but does not further sensitize FA-C mutant cells suggesting they are already fully compromised.[98] Interestingly, the ability of FANCC to inhibit the kinase activity of PKR is independent of the ability of FANCC to interact with other FA proteins.[99]

Surprisingly, given this involvement of FANCC in cytokine signaling pathways, in vivo administration of IFN-γ to *Fancc-/-* mice with and without subsequent Fas-ligation, did not induce bone marrow failure as shown by lack of effect on blood counts, progenitor colony formation and marrow cellularity.[100]

FANCC in DNA Damage and Repair

The much lower doses of MMC required to generate an equivalent amount of DNA interstrand crosslinks (ICLs) in FA-C cells compared to corrected isogenic counterparts and nonFA cells suggests a pre-repair defect. The efficiency of ICL repair in corrected FA-C, normal and mock transfected FA-C LCLs differentially treated to generate similar levels of ICL damage is similar, suggesting repair is not affected by the presence of FANCC.[36]

Other studies have implicated FANCC in the repair of specific types of DNA damage. A plasmid-based DNA end-joining assay in FA-C LCLs revealed that error-free processing of blunt-ended DSB is greatly reduced, resulting in both increased frequency and size of deletions. Complementation with *FANCC* cDNA restores fidelity of this blunt-ended DSB processing.[101] An FA-C LCL has also been shown to repair the oxidative DNA damage in plasmid DNA extracellularly treated with potassium permanganate less efficiently than did nonFA cells, and this defect is also complemented by exogenous expression of FANCC.[102]

FA-C LCLs, as well as cells from other FA subtypes, are unable to activate the assembly of RMN complex proteins (RAD50/MRE11/NBS1) into subnuclear foci in response to ICL inducers. DSB formation and unhooking of ICLs in response to MMC is normal, indicating that absence of RMN assembly is not simply due to absence of DNA ends produced as intermediates of crosslinking. MMC treatment induces phosphorylation of NBS1 in corrected cells, but not in FA-C cells. Notably, phosphorylated NBS1 participates in activation of DNA-damage dependent S-phase arrest and FA cells are deficient in ICL-dependent S-phase checkpoint activation.[65] In contrast, formation of RMN foci and phosphorylation of NBS-1 in response to ionizing radiation was normal in FA cells.[103]

On exposure to MMC, Rad51 foci formation in normal and corrected FA-C LCLs increases; however, in uncorrected FA-C cells this response is reduced and delayed, despite normal levels of Rad51 protein. BRCA1 foci formation is also delayed in response to MMC treatment in FA-C cells. Rad51 foci formation in response to gamma-irradiation was normal in FA-C LCLs,[103] although another study using primary fibroblasts found significantly reduced Rad51 foci formation in response to ionizing radiation.[104]

FANCC and Oxidative Stress

At ambient 20% oxygen, when MMC is expected to generate free radicals through redox cycling, FA-C LCLs increase induction of apoptosis in response to low-dose MMC. In contrast, at hypoxic 5% oxygen, when the metabolic activation of MMC for crosslinking is facilitated, levels of apoptosis observed are not different from normal cells.[105]

FANCC binds to NADPH: cytochrome c (P450) reductase (RED), a microsomal membrane protein involved in electron transfer, including the bioreductive activation of MMC. The interaction, which involves the cytosolic membrane proximal domain of the reductase that contains a flavin mononucleotide (FMN) binding site, is disrupted by addition of FMN to lysates. The catalytic activity of RED is attenuated by overexpression of FANCC, but cannot be suppressed completely. Thus a role for FANCC in fine-tuning of the redox state of cell has been proposed.[106]

Association of FANCC with glutathione S-transferase P1-1 (GSTP1) increases GSTP1 activity in murine haematopoietic cells particularly after induction of apoptosis by factor withdrawal. FANCC functions by preventing the formation of inactivating disulphide bonds within GST during apoptosis.[107] FANCC overexpression attenuates glutathione (GSH) depletion after apoptotic induction, and if GSH is artificially depleted the antiapoptotic effect of GSTP1 appears dependent on total amount FANCC available to keep it in reduced state. The eight cysteine residues conserved in FANCC across species [12] have been proposed as possible participants in thiol-disulphide exchange.[107]

In vivo alteration of redox state in *Fancc-/-* mice was suggested by the result of a cross to mice with targeted mutagenesis of the Cu/Zn superoxide dismutase gene (*Sod1*). Although not displaying developmental defects or increased chromosomal aberrations typical of FA, *Fancc-/-Sod1-/-* mice had a phenotype of bone marrow hypocellularity with bicytopaenia. Absolute numbers of primitive haematopoeitic progenitors was similar to normal but a decrease in committed progenitor populations was demonstrated by severely reduced in vitro clonogenic potential of committed myeloid and lymphoid progenitors compared to *Fancc-/-* and *Sod-/-* null mutants.[108]

A link between reactive oxygen species (ROS) induction and Fas-priming by IFN has been suggested by increased ROS accumulation and decreased intracellular glutathione levels in FA-C LCLs primed with IFN-γ and treated with Fas-agonist antibody compared to isogenic corrected cells. The antioxidant dehydroascorbic acid (DHA) reduced the Fas-priming effect of IFN-γ confirming ROS as a mediator of the exaggerated IFN-γ response.[109] IFN-γ induced ROS accumulation in FA-C LCLs is accompanied by activation of the stress-activated protein kinases JNK and p38 and prevention of the stress kinase activation by DHA implies it is due to ROS. Partial inhibition of caspase-3 activation by inhibitors of p38 but not JNK suggests IFN-γ and Fas ligation can mediate signals for apoptosis in FA-C cells via p38 but that other pathways must also be involved. Hydrogen peroxide exposure also results in ROS accumulation with p38 and JNK activation in FA-C cell lines, but not in corrected cells or in uncorrected FA-C cells pretreated with DHA.[110]

Nitric oxide (NO) is also a factor in the sensitivity of *Fancc-/-* bone marrow progenitor cells to cytokines. In vitro cytokine-mediated growth inhibition of *Fancc-/-* bone marrow progenitor cells is prevented by inhibition of NO synthase activity, whereas growth inhibition by two different NO-generating agents is greater in *Fancc-/-* haematopoeitic cells than in wild type cells. Furthermore, stimulation of *Fancc-/-* bone marrow-derived macrophages with IFN-γ and bacterial lipopolysaccharide results in increased inducible nitric oxide synthase (iNOS) levels and increased nitrite release.[111]

Fancc-/- HPCs and MEFs are highly sensitive to oxidant stimuli as shown by clonogenic progenitor assays of cells exposed to hydrogen peroxide (H_2O_2). Oxidant-mediated apoptosis is increased in *Fancc-/-* MEFs and treatment of these MEFs with anti-oxidants before culture with H_2O_2 reduces apoptosis and returns survival to wild type levels.[112] The serine-threonine kinase apoptosis signal-regulating kinase 1 (ASK1), a MAPKKK able to activate the JNK and p38 signalling cascades[113] active in FA-C LCLs treated with H_2O_2 or IFN-γ and Fas ligation,[110] is hyperactivated in H_2O_2-treated *Fancc-/-* MEFs. Inhibition of ASK1 activity by a dominant negative ASK1 mutant, or reduction of ASK1 expression by siRNA alleviated H_2O_2 induced apoptosis, suggesting it is ASK1 dependent. Transduction of FANCC-E251A has the same protective effect on viability of *Fancc-/-* MEFs as wild-type FANCC, whereas FANCC-322delG gave no protection against H_2O_2. This implies the role of FANCC in HSP70/PKR signaling is not required for the protective effect, another example of the multiplicity of FANCC function.[112]

Conclusions

The understanding of FANCC protein function has improved considerably since the initial discovery that loss of function of a previously unknown protein with no obvious functional motifs was causal in the FA-C defect. The generation of isogenic LCLs with and without FANCC expression has allowed controlled examination of many aspects of the FA cellular phenotype. Discoveries such as the defect in arrest of S-phase replication [65] and the altered behaviour of the RMN complex proteins in response to ICL-inducers,[103] have provided important clues to FANCC function in mediating cellular response to DNA-damaging agents. The generation of *Fancc-/-* mice has also been invaluable, allowing the use of primary non-immortalized cellular materials that are rarely, if ever, available from patients, and making it possible to perform in vivo studies of haematopoiesis.

Although the number of possible cellular roles for FANCC seems ever-increasing, new discoveries often link back to previous findings and recurrent themes have emerged. The recent demonstration of the cooperativity of p53 and FANCC in suppression of tumorigenesis[70] is interesting given that p53 can be activated by PKR,[114] which is in turn inhibited by FANCC interaction with HSP70.[99] The ASK1 apoptotic program, observed in *Fancc-/-* MEFs treated with H_2O_2,[112] is known to be initiated when redox sensitive proteins that bind to and inactivate ASK1 become oxidated and dissociate. Among these redox sensitive proteins are the GSTs,[115,116] at least one class of which, GSTP1, is maintained in a reduced state by FANCC.[107]

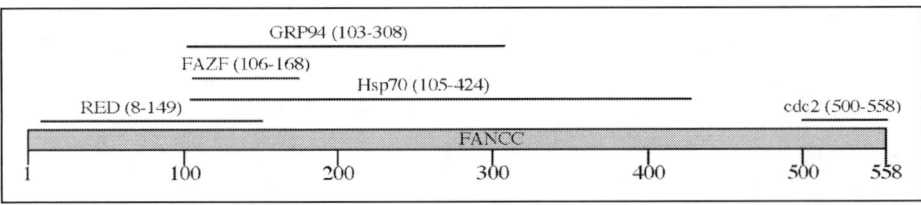

Figure 3. Amino acid residues in FANCC identified as critical for direct and indirect protein interactions. FANCC residues implicated in binding are indicated in brackets beside the name of the interacting protein. In the case of other interacting proteins, either no subregion of FANCC independently able to mediate the interaction was identified (e.g., FANCE), or no mapping of regions involved in interaction was performed (e.g., GSTP1).

Even as discoveries seem to connect together, some diversity in FANCC function is suggested by the multiple subcellular localizations of the protein, as well as overlap in the residues of FANCC critical for mediating different protein-protein interactions (Fig. 3). Multiplicity of function is also demonstrated by the differential ability of certain FANCC mutants to correct FA-C cellular phenotypes such as MMC sensitivity, failure of FA protein complex formation, lack of STAT1 activation, hyperactivation of PKR, and elevated ASK1-mediated apoptosis. This finding is of particular interest in the assessment of genotype-phenotype correlations. For example, the M55 mutant found in FA-C cells with a 322delG mutation allows for normal STAT1 activation, which may help to account for the relatively mild phenotype seen in these patients.[96] Of equal interest is that the converse may also be true. Although FANCC mutants that prevent HSP70 interaction but correct MMC sensitivity have so far been artificially generated in alanine mutagenesis studies, the possibility that such mutations exist in nature, but have not yet been discovered due to failure to produce a classical FA phenotype, is very real. Testing of *FANCC* variants identified in sporadic cancers[31,117] may be of particular interest in this regard.

Studies of FANCC expression, subcellular localization, protein interactions, and gain and loss of function have demonstrated roles for FANCC in a wide range of cellular activities, some of which may be interconnected. One major role for FANCC is cooperation with other FA proteins in a protein complex in both the nuclear and cytoplasmic compartments. Other largely cytoplasmic roles may be unique to FANCC, including protection against the cytotoxicity of IFN-γ and TNFα via association with HSP70 and PKR, and maintenance of the redox state of the cell via interactions with RED and GSTP1. Defects in the differentiation and proliferation of HPCs and germ cells seen with *Fancc* loss of function may be mediated by both nuclear and cytoplasmic activities of the FANCC protein.

Acknowledgments

Work in our laboratory has been supported by the Canadian Institutes of Health Research (CIHR) and the Hospital for Sick Children Foundation. MB holds the Lombard Insurance Chair in Pediatric Research, Hospital for Sick Children and University of Toronto.

References

1. Strathdee CA, Gavish H, Shannon WR et al. Cloning of cDNAs for Fanconi's anaemia by functional complementation. Nature 1992; 358:434.
2. Joenje H, Patel KJ. The emerging genetic and molecular basis of Fanconi anaemia. Nat Rev Genet 2001; 2:446-57.
3. Strathdee CA, Duncan AM, Buchwald M. Evidence for at least four Fanconi anaemia genes including FACC on chromosome 9. Nat Genet 1992; 1:196-8.
4. Morris DJ, Reis A. A YAC contig spanning the nevoid basal cell carcinoma syndrome, Fanconi anaemia group C, and xeroderma pigmentosum group A loci on chromosome 9q. Genomics 1994; 23:23-9.
5. Gibson RA, Buchwald M, Roberts RG et al. Characterisation of the exon structure of the Fanconi anaemia group C gene by vectorette PCR. Hum Mol Genet 1993; 2:35-8.
6. Gibson RA, Hajianpour A, Murer-Orlando M et al. A nonsense mutation and exon skipping in the Fanconi anaemia group C gene. Hum Mol Genet 1993; 2:797-9.
7. Savoia A, Centra M, Ianzano L et al. Characterization of the 5' region of the Fanconi anaemia group C (FACC) gene. Hum Mol Genet 1995; 4:1321-6.
8. Tower PA, Christianson TA, Peters ST et al. Expression of the Fanconi anemia group C gene in hematopoietic cells is not influenced by oxidative stress, cross-linking agents, radiation, heat, or mitotic inhibitory factors. Exp Hematol 1998; 26:19-26.
9. Liebetrau W, Budde A, Savoia A et al. p53 activates Fanconi anemia group C gene expression. Hum Mol Genet 1997; 6:277-83.
10. Wevrick R, Clarke CA, Buchwald M. Cloning and analysis of the murine Fanconi anemia group C cDNA. Hum Mol Genet 1993; 2:655-62.
11. Wevrick R, Barker JE, Nadeau JH et al. Mapping of the murine and rat Facc genes and assessment of flexed-tail as a candidate mouse homolog of Fanconi anemia group C. Mamm Genome 1993; 4:440-4.

12. Wong JCY, Alon N, Buchwald M. Cloning of the bovine and rat Fanconi anemia group C cDNA. Mamm Genome 1997; 8:522-5.
13. Yamashita T, Kupfer GM, Naf D et al. The Fanconi anemia pathway requires FAA phosphorylation and FAA/FAC nuclear accumulation. Proc Natl Acad Sci USA 1998; 95:13085-90.
14. Parker L, dos Santos C, Buchwald M. The delta327 mutation in the Fanconi anemia group C gene generates a novel transcript lacking the first two coding exons. Hum Mutat 1998; Suppl:S275-7.
15. Murer-Orlando M, Llerena JC, Jr., Birjandi F et al. FACC gene mutations and early prenatal diagnosis of Fanconi's anaemia. Lancet 1993 342:686.
16. Gibson RA, Morgan NV, Goldstein LH et al. Novel mutations and polymorphisms in the Fanconi anemia group C gene. Hum Mutat 1996; 8:140-8.
17. Whitney MA, Saito H, Jakobs PM et al. A common mutation in the FACC gene causes Fanconi anaemia in Ashkenazi Jews. Nat Genet 1993; 4:202-5.
18. Lo Ten Foe JR, Kruyt FA, Zweekhorst MB et al. Exon 6 skipping in the Fanconi anemia C gene associated with a nonsense/missense mutation (775C->T) in exon 5: the first example of a nonsense mutation in one exon causing skipping of another downstream. Hum Mutat 1998; Suppl:S25-7.
19. Lo Ten Foe JR, Rooimans MA, Joenje H, Arwert F. Novel frameshift mutation (1806insA) in exon 14 of the Fanconi anemia C gene, FAC. Hum Mutat 1996; 7:264-5.
20. Lo ten Foe JR, Barel MT, Thuss P et al. Sequence variations in the Fanconi anaemia gene, FAC: pathogenicity of 1806insA and R548X and recognition of D195V as a polymorphic variant. Hum Genet 1996; 98:522-3.
21. Waisfisz Q, Morgan NV, Savino M et al. Spontaneous functional correction of homozygous fanconi anaemia alleles reveals novel mechanistic basis for reverse mosaicism. Nat Genet 1999; 22:379-83.
22. Gavish H, dos Santos CC, Buchwald M. A Leu554-to-Pro substitution completely abolishes the functional complementing activity of the Fanconi anemia (FACC) protein. Hum Mol Genet 1993; 2:123-6.
23. Youssoufian H, Li Y, Martin ME et al. Induction of Fanconi anemia cellular phenotype in human 293 cells by overexpression of a mutant FAC allele. J Clin Invest 1996; 97:957-62.
24. Gibson RA, Ford D, Jansen S et al. Genetic mapping of the FACC gene and linkage analysis in Fanconi anaemia families. J Med Genet 1994; 31:868-71.
25. Verlander PC, Lin JD, Udono MU et al. Mutation analysis of the Fanconi anemia gene FACC. Am J Hum Genet 1994; 54:595-601.
26. Faivre L, Guardiola P, Lewis C et al. Association of complementation group and mutation type with clinical outcome in fanconi anemia. European Fanconi Anemia Research Group. Blood 2000; 96:4064-70.
27. Yamashita T, Wu N, Kupfer G et al. Clinical variability of Fanconi anemia (type C) results from expression of an amino terminal truncated Fanconi anemia complementation group C polypeptide with partial activity. Blood 1996; 87:4424-32.
28. Futaki M, Yamashita T, Yagasaki H et al. The IVS4 + 4 A to T mutation of the fanconi anemia gene FANCC is not associated with a severe phenotype in Japanese patients. Blood 2000; 95:1493-8.
29. Seal S, Barfoot R, Jayatilake H et al. Evaluation of Fanconi Anemia genes in familial breast cancer predisposition. Cancer Res 2003;63:8596-9.
30. Awan A, Malcolm Taylor G, Gokhale DA et al. Increased frequency of Fanconi anemia group C genetic variants in children with sporadic acute myeloid leukemia [letter]. Blood 1998; 91:4813-4.
31. van der Heijden MS, Yeo CJ, Hruban RH et al. Fanconi anemia gene mutations in young-onset pancreatic cancer. Cancer Res 2003; 63:2585-8.
32. Rischewski JR, Clausen H, Leber V et al. A heterozygous frameshift mutation in the Fanconi anemia C gene in familial T-ALL and secondary malignancy. Klin Padiatr 2000; 212:174-6.
33. Krasnoshtein F, Buchwald M. Developmental expression of the Fac gene correlates with congenital defects in Fanconi anemia patients. Hum Mol Genet 1996; 5:85-93.
34. Brady G, Billia F, Knox J et al. Analysis of gene expression in a complex differentiation hierarchy by global amplification of cDNA from single cells. Curr Biol 1995; 5:909-22.
35. Aube M, Lafrance M, Brodeur I et al. Fanconi anemia genes are highly expressed in primitive CD34+ hematopoietic cells. BMC Blood Disord 2003; 3:1.
36. Youssoufian H. Cytoplasmic localization of FAC is essential for the correction of a prerepair defect in Fanconi anemia group C cells. J Clin Invest 1996; 97:2003-10.
37. Joenje H, Youssoufian H, Kruyt FA et al. Expression of the Fanconi anemia gene FAC in human cell lines: lack of effect of oxygen tension. Blood Cells Mol Dis 1995; 21:182-91.
38. Heinrich MC, Silvey KV, Stone S et al. Posttranscriptional cell cycle-dependent regulation of human FANCC expression. Blood 2000; 95:3970-7.

39. Kupfer GM, Yamashita T, Naf D et al. The Fanconi anemia polypeptide, FAC, binds to the cyclin-dependent kinase, cdc2. Blood 1997; 90:1047-54.
40. Brodeur I, Goulet I, Tremblay CS et al. Regulation of the Fanconi anemia group C protein through proteolytic modification. J Biol Chem 2004; 279:4713-20.
41. Hoshino T, Wang J, Devetten MP et al. Molecular chaperone GRP94 binds to the Fanconi anemia group C protein and regulates its intracellular expression. Blood 1998; 91:4379-86.
42. Youssoufian H. Localization of Fanconi anemia C protein to the cytoplasm of mammalian cells. Proc Natl Acad Sci USA 1994; 91:7975-9.
43. Yamashita T, Barber DL, Zhu Y et al. The Fanconi anemia polypeptide FACC is localized to the cytoplasm. Proc Natl Acad Sci USA 1994 ;91:6712-6.
44. Youssoufian H, Auerbach AD, Verlander PC et al. Identification of cytosolic proteins that bind to the Fanconi anemia complementation group C polypeptide in vitro. Evidence for a multimeric complex. J Biol Chem 1995; 270:9876-82.
45. Hoatlin ME, Christianson TA, Keeble WW et al. The Fanconi anemia group C gene product is located in both the nucleus and cytoplasm of human cells. Blood 1998; 91:1418-25.
46. Savoia A, Garcia-Higuera I, D'Andrea AD. Nuclear localization of the Fanconi anemia protein FANCC is required for functional activity [letter]. Blood 1999; 93:4025-6.
47. Hoatlin ME, Zhi Y, Ball H et al. A novel BTB/POZ transcriptional repressor protein interacts with the Fanconi anemia group C protein and PLZF. Blood 1999; 94:3737-47.
48. Pace P, Johnson M, Tan WM et al. FANCE: the link between Fanconi anaemia complex assembly and activity. Embo J 2002; 21:3414-23.
49. de Winter JP, Leveille F, van Berkel CG et al. Isolation of a cDNA representing the Fanconi anemia complementation group E gene. Am J Hum Genet 2000; 67:1306-8.
50. Medhurst AL, Huber PA, Waisfisz Q et al. Direct interactions of the five known Fanconi anaemia proteins suggest a common functional pathway. Hum Mol Genet 2001; 10:423-9.
51. Gordon SM, Buchwald M. Fanconi anemia protein complex: mapping protein interactions in the yeast 2- and 3-hybrid systems. Blood 2003; 102:136-41.
52. Taniguchi T, D'Andrea AD. The Fanconi anemia protein, FANCE, promotes the nuclear accumulation of FANCC. Blood 2002; 100:2457-62.
53. Garcia-Higuera I, Taniguchi T, Ganesan S et al. Interaction of the Fanconi anemia proteins and BRCA1 in a common pathway. Mol Cell 2001; 7:249-62.
54. Kupfer GM, Naf D, Suliman A et al. The Fanconi anaemia proteins, FAA and FAC, interact to form a nuclear complex. Nat Genet 1997; 17:487-90.
55. Garcia-Higuera I, Kuang Y, Naf D et al. Fanconi anemia proteins FANCA, FANCC, and FANCG/XRCC9 interact in a functional nuclear complex. Mol Cell Biol 1999; 19:4866-73.
56. de Winter JP, van der Weel L, de Groot J et al. The Fanconi anemia protein FANCF forms a nuclear complex with FANCA, FANCC and FANCG. Hum Mol Genet 2000; 9:2665-74.
57. Meetei AR, de Winter JP, Medhurst AL et al. A novel ubiquitin ligase is deficient in Fanconi anemia. Nat Genet 2003; 35:165-70.
58. Thomashevski A, High AA, Drozd M et al. The fanconi anemia core complex forms 4 different sized complexes in different subcellular compartments. J Biol Chem 2004; 13:13.
59. Qiao F, Moss A, Kupfer GM. Fanconi anemia proteins localize to chromatin and the nuclear matrix in a DNA damage- and cell cycle-regulated manner. J Biol Chem 2001; 276:23391-6.
60. McMahon LW, Sangerman J, Goodman SR et al. Human alpha spectrin II and the FANCA, FANCC, and FANCG proteins bind to DNA containing psoralen interstrand cross-links. Biochemistry 2001; 40:7025-7034.
61. Barna M, Merghoub T, Costoya JA et al. Plzf mediates transcriptional repression of HoxD gene expression through chromatin remodeling. Dev Cell 2002; 3:499-510.
62. Dai MS, Chevallier N, Stone S et al. The effects of the Fanconi anemia zinc finger (FAZF) on cell cycle, apoptosis, and proliferation are differentiation stage-specific. J Biol Chem 2002; 277:26327-34.
63. Kruyt FA, Dijkmans LM, Arwert F et al. Involvement of the Fanconi's anemia protein FAC in a pathway that signals to the cyclin B/cdc2 kinase. Cancer Res 1997; 57:2244-51.
64. Heinrich MC, Hoatlin ME, Zigler AJ et al. DNA cross-linker-induced G2/M arrest in group C Fanconi anemia lymphoblasts reflects normal checkpoint function. Blood 1998; 91:275-87.
65. Sala-Trepat M, Rouillard D, Escarceller M et al. Arrest of S-phase progression is impaired in Fanconi anemia cells. Exp Cell Res 2000; 260:208-15.
66. Akkari YM, Bateman RL, Reifsteck CA et al. The 4N cell cycle delay in Fanconi anemia reflects growth arrest in late S phase. Mol Genet Metab 2001;74:403-12.
67. Kupfer GM, D'Andrea AD. The effect of the Fanconi anemia polypeptide, FAC, upon p53 induction and G2 checkpoint regulation. Blood 1996; 88:1019-25.

68. Marathi UK, Howell SR, Ashmun RA et al. The Fanconi anemia complementation group C protein corrects DNA interstrand cross-link-specific apoptosis in HSC536N cells. Blood 1996; 88:2298-305.
69. Kruyt FA, Dijkmans LM, van den Berg TK et al. Fanconi anemia genes act to suppress a cross-linker-inducible p53- independent apoptosis pathway in lymphoblastoid cell lines. Blood 1996; 87:938-48.
70. Freie B, Li X, Ciccone SL, et al. Fanconi anemia type C and p53 cooperate in apoptosis and tumorigenesis. Blood 2003; 102:4146-52.
71. Ridet A, Guillouf C, Duchaud E et al. Deregulated apoptosis is a hallmark of the Fanconi anemia syndrome. Cancer Res 1997; 57:1722-30.
72. Guillouf C, Vit JP, Rosselli F. Loss of the Fanconi anemia group C protein activity results in an inability to activate caspase-3 after ionizing radiation. Biochimie 2000; 82:51-8.
73. Clarke AA, Gibson FM, Scott J et al. Fanconi's anemia cell lines show distinct mechanisms of cell death in response to mitomycin C or agonistic anti-Fas antibodies. Haematologica 2004; 89:11-20.
74. Segal GM, Magenis RE, Brown M et al. Repression of Fanconi anemia gene (FACC) expression inhibits growth of hematopoietic progenitor cells. J Clin Invest 1994; 94:846-52.
75. Chen M, Tomkins DJ, Auerbach W, et al. Inactivation of Fac in mice produces inducible chromosomal instability and reduced fertility reminiscent of Fanconi anaemia. Nat Genet 1996; 12:448-51.
76. Whitney MA, Royle G, Low MJ et al. Germ cell defects and hematopoietic hypersensitivity to gamma- interferon in mice with a targeted disruption of the Fanconi anemia C gene. Blood 1996; 88:49-58.
77. Tomkins DJ, Care M, Carreau M et al. Development and characterization of immortalized fibroblastoid cell lines from an FA(C) mouse model. Mutat Res 1998; 408:27-35.
78. Otsuki T, Wang J, Demuth I et al. Assessment of mitomycin C sensitivity in Fanconi anemia complementation group C gene (Fac) knock-out mouse cells. Int J Hematol 1998; 67:243-8.
79. Nadler JJ, Braun RE. Fanconi anemia complementation group C is required for proliferation of murine primordial germ cells. Genesis 2000; 27:117-23.
80. Haneline LS, Broxmeyer HE, Cooper S et al. Multiple inhibitory cytokines induce deregulated progenitor growth and apoptosis in hematopoietic cells from Fac-/- mice. Blood 1998; 91:4092-8.
81. Haneline LS, Gobbett TA, Ramani R et al. Loss of FancC function results in decreased hematopoietic stem cell repopulating ability. Blood 1999; 94:1-8.
82. Carreau M, Gan OI, Liu L et al. Hematopoietic compartment of Fanconi anemia group C null mice contains fewer lineage-negative CD34+ primitive hematopoietic cells and shows reduced reconstruction ability. Exp Hematol 1999; 27:1667-74.
83. Aube M, Lafrance M, Charbonneau C et al. Hematopoietic stem cells from fancc(-/-) mice have lower growth and differentiation potential in response to growth factors. Stem Cells 2002; 20:438-47.
84. Otsuki T, Nagakura S, Wang J et al. Tumor necrosis factor-alpha and CD95 ligation suppress erythropoiesis in Fanconi anemia C gene knockout mice. J Cell Physiol 1999; 179:79-86.
85. Haneline LS, Li X, Ciccone SL et al. Retroviral-mediated expression of recombinant Fancc enhances the repopulating ability of Fancc-/- hematopoietic stem cells and decreases the risk of clonal evolution. Blood. 2003; 101:1299-1307.
86. Carreau M, Gan OI, Liu L et al. Bone marrow failure in the Fanconi anemia group C mouse model after DNA damage. Blood 1998; 91:2737-2744.
87. Gush KA, Fu KL, Grompe M et al. Phenotypic correction of Fanconi anemia group C knockout mice. Blood 2000; 95:700-4.
88. Cumming RC, Liu JM, Youssoufian H et al. Suppression of apoptosis in hematopoietic factor-dependent progenitor cell lines by expression of the FAC gene. Blood. 1996; 88:4558-67.
89. Wang J, Otsuki T, Youssoufian H et al. Overexpression of the fanconi anemia group C gene (FAC) protects hematopoietic progenitors from death induced by Fas-mediated apoptosis. Cancer Res 1998; 58:3538-41.
90. Rathbun RK, Faulkner GR, Ostroski MH et al. Inactivation of the Fanconi anemia group C gene augments interferon-gamma-induced apoptotic responses in hematopoietic cells. Blood 1997; 90:974-985.
91. Koh PS, Hughes GC, Faulkner GR et al. The Fanconi anemia group C gene product modulates apoptotic responses to tumor necrosis factor-alpha and Fas ligand but does not suppress expression of receptors of the tumor necrosis factor receptor superfamily. Exp Hematol 1999; 27:1-8.
92. Rathbun RK, Christianson TA, Faulkner GR et al. Interferon-gamma-induced apoptotic responses of Fanconi anemia group C hematopoietic progenitor cells involve caspase 8-dependent activation of caspase 3 family members. Blood 2000; 96:4204-11.

93. Rutherford TR, Myatt NE, Gibson FM et al. The Fanconi anemia cell line HSC536N is not sensitive to interferon- gamma and does not cleave PARP in response to FAS-mediated cell killing. Blood 2002; 99:2627-8; discussion 2629-30.
94. Pang Q, Fagerlie S, Christianson TA et al. The Fanconi anemia protein FANCC binds to and facilitates the activation of STAT1 by gamma interferon and hematopoietic growth factors. Mol Cell Biol 2000; 20:4724-35.
95. Fagerlie S, Lensch MW, Pang Q et al. The Fanconi anemia group C gene product: signaling functions in hematopoietic cells. Exp Hematol 2001; 29:1371-81.
96. Pang Q, Christianson TA, Keeble W et al. The Fanconi anemia complementation group C gene product: structural evidence of multifunctionality. Blood 2001; 98:1392-401.
97. Pang Q, Keeble W, Diaz J et al. Role of double-stranded RNA-dependent protein kinase in mediating hypersensitivity of Fanconi anemia complementation group C cells to interferon gamma, tumor necrosis factor-alpha, and double-stranded RNA. Blood 2001; 97:1644-52.
98. Pang Q, Keeble W, Christianson TA et al. FANCC interacts with Hsp70 to protect hematopoietic cells from IFN- gamma/TNF-alpha-mediated cytotoxicity. Embo J 2001; 20:4478-89.
99. Pang Q, Christianson TA, Keeble W et al. The anti-apoptotic function of Hsp70 in the interferon-inducible double-stranded RNA-dependent protein kinase-mediated death signaling pathway requires the Fanconi anemia protein, FANCC. J Biol Chem 2002; 277:49638-43.
100. Kurre P, Anandakumar P, Grompe M et al. In vivo administration of interferon gamma does not cause marrow aplasia in mice with a targeted disruption of FANCC. Exp Hematol 2002; 30:1257-62.
101. Escarceller M, Buchwald M, Singleton BK et al. Fanconi anemia C gene product plays a role in the fidelity of blunt DNA end-joining. J Mol Biol. 1998; 279:375-85.
102. Lackinger D, Ruppitsch W, Ramirez MH et al. Involvement of the Fanconi anemia protein FA-C in repair processes of oxidative DNA damages. FEBS Lett 1998; 440:103-6.
103. Pichierri P, Averbeck D, Rosselli F. DNA cross-link-dependent RAD50/MRE11/NBS1 subnuclear assembly requires the Fanconi anemia C protein. Hum Mol Genet 2002; 11:2531-46.
104. Digweed M, Rothe S, Demuth I et al. Attenuation of the formation of DNA-repair foci containing RAD51 in Fanconi anaemia. Carcinogenesis 2002; 23:1121-6.
105. Clarke AA, Philpott NJ, Gordon-Smith EC et al. The sensitivity of Fanconi anaemia group C cells to apoptosis induced by mitomycin C is due to oxygen radical generation, not DNA crosslinking. Br J Haematol. 1997; 96:240-7.
106. Kruyt FA, Hoshino T, Liu JM et al. Abnormal microsomal detoxification implicated in Fanconi anemia group C by interaction of the FAC protein with NADPH cytochrome P450 reductase. Blood 1998; 92:3050-6.
107. Cumming RC, Lightfoot J, Beard K et al. Fanconi anemia group C protein prevents apoptosis in hematopoietic cells through redox regulation of GSTP1. Nat Med 2001; 7:814-20.
108. Hadjur S, Ung K, Wadsworth L et al. Defective hematopoiesis and hepatic steatosis in mice with combined deficiencies of the genes encoding Fancc and Cu/Zn superoxide dismutase. Blood 2001; 98:1003-11.
109. Pearl-Yafe M, Halperin D, Halevy A et al. An oxidative mechanism of interferon induced priming of the Fas pathway in Fanconi anemia cells. Biochem Pharmacol. 2003; 65:833-42.
110. Pearl-Yafe M, Halperin D, Scheuerman O et al. The p38 pathway partially mediates caspase-3 activation induced by reactive oxygen species in Fanconi anemia C cells. Biochem Pharmacol 2004; 67:539-46.
111. Hadjur S, Jirik FR. Increased sensitivity of Fancc-deficient hematopoietic cells to nitric oxide and evidence that this species mediates growth inhibition by cytokines. Blood 2003;101:3877-84
112. Saadatzadeh MR, Bijangi-Vishehsaraei K, Hong P et al. Oxidant Hypersensitivity of Fanconi Anemia Type C-deficient Cells Is Dependent on a Redox-regulated Apoptotic Pathway. J Biol Chem 2004; 279:16805-12.
113. Takeda K, Matsuzawa A, Nishitoh H et al. Roles of MAPKKK ASK1 in stress-induced cell death. Cell Struct Funct 2003; 28:23-9.
114. Cuddihy AR, Wong AH, Tam NW et al. The double-stranded RNA activated protein kinase PKR physically associates with the tumor suppressor p53 protein and phosphorylates human p53 on serine 392 in vitro. Oncogene 1999; 18:2690-702.
115. Cho SG, Lee YH, Park HS et al. Glutathione S-transferase mu modulates the stress-activated signals by suppressing apoptosis signal-regulating kinase 1. J Biol Chem 2001; 276:12749-55.
116. Gilot D, Loyer P, Corlu A, et al. Liver protection from apoptosis requires both blockage of initiator caspase activities and inhibition of ASK1/JNK pathway via glutathione S-transferase regulation. J Biol Chem 2002; 277:49220-9.
117. Barber LM, McGrath HE, Meyer S, et al. Constitutional sequence variation in the Fanconi anaemia group C (FANCC) gene in childhood acute myeloid leukaemia. Br J Haematol 2003; 121:57-62.

CHAPTER 5

The *FANC B, E, F* and *G* Genes and Their Products

Filippo Rosselli*

The rare autosomal recessive syndrome Fanconi anemia (FA) leads to bone marrow failure and malignancy predisposition. Moreover, patients may present with several con-genital anomalies of the skeleton and genito-urinary tract, growth retardation and hyperpigmentation of the skin. Cells from FA patients are hypersensitive to crosslinking agents, and this hypersensitivity is the basis for a diagnostic test as well as enabling exploration of the genetic heterogeneity of the disease.[1,2,50,58]

Starting with the considerable variation observed at both clinical and cellular level in FA syndrome, the presence of an underlying genetic heterogeneity was suspected. The existence of at least two complementation groups, named A and NonA, was determined by testing for complementation of the cellular and chromosomal hypersensitivity to mitomycin C in somatic cell hybrids constructed with lymphoblasts derived from four different FA patients.[10] Since that time, the number of FA complementation groups increased to four in 1992,[54] concomitant with the cloning of the first, FANCC,[55] to eight in 1997[28] and it is presently 12.[33] FA-A is the most common FA subtype, accounting for about 65% of the affected individuals, FA-C and FA-G each represent less than 15% of the cases, the other groups being extremely rare. The genes coding for the groups A, C, D1, D2, E, F, G and L have been cloned using several strategies, including functional cloning, chromosome walking, reverse genetics and direct sequencing of a potential gene.[7-9,25,35,36,45,55,57] Complementation analysis and gene cloning, leading to the discovery of the pathological mutations of *FANCC* genes, opened the possibility of determining the genotype/phenotype relationships and establishing a link between complementation group and the clinical outcome or the degree of hypersensitivity to cross-linking agent treatment. Although the diversity of the clinical traits is insufficient to class a patient in a defined complementation group, some significant differences have been reported in a large study that analyzed 245 FA patients from FA-A to FA-G complementation groups as well as mutations in *FANCA* and *FANCC* genes. The results of that analysis indicated that (1) FA-G patients had a more severe pancytopenia and a higher risk of leukemia, (2) FA-D, FA-E and FA-F patients showed more somatic anomalies touching several different anatomic sites, including the head, the skeleton, the kidneys, the urogenital trait, the cardiovascular and central nervous systems, and (3) FA-A patients homozygous for null mutations presented earlier onset of anemia.[14]

The cloning of *FANCC*, the first identified FA gene, closed a period during which the studies on FA essentially provided information concerning the phenotypic traits of the syndrome, at both clinical and cellular levels. The gene cloning opened the possibility to shed light on the molecular process(es) responsible for FA phenotypic heterogeneity.[55] Unfortunately, the

---

*Filippo Rosselli—Laboratory of Genetic Stability and Cancer, UPR 2169, CNRS, Gustave Roussy Institute PR2, 39, Rue Camille Desmoulins, 94805 Villejuif, France. Email: Rosselli@igr.fr

Molecular Mechanisms of Fanconi Anemia, edited by Shamim I. Ahmad and Sandra H. Kirk. ©2006 Eurekah.com and Springer Science+Business Media.

sequences of most of the cloned genes failed to reveal major structural or functional domains in the predicted FA proteins. The different FA gene products failed to share significant similarity to each other or with other proteins. For these reasons, the identification of the genes was not followed by a rapid understanding of the functions of their products.

The studies carried out between the end of the 70's and the beginning of the 90's have been identified three major biological end-points as altered in FA: (a) the cellular and chromosomal responses to cross-linking agents exposure; (b) the process of detoxification or production of toxic free radicals; and (c) the production or the cellular and molecular responses to pleiotropic cytokines involved in hematopoiesis, stress responses and cancer.[4] Anomalies were observed in that physiological clues indicate an involvement of FANC proteins in DNA repair/cell cycle checkpoints, detoxification and differentiation processes.

Several recent works clearly identified that DNA damage is a major signal in activation of the FANC proteins and that the DNA repair/cell cycle checkpoint function is a main pathway requiring FANC protein activities.[6,50,59] Nevertheless, on the basis of functional and physical interactions, an involvement in free radical metabolism was also inferred.[5,16,24,30,40] Finally, it appears that, at least in the absence of DNA damage induced by exogenous agents, FA gene products are also involved in cytokine signalling/metabolism. This function could be involved in the abnormalities observed in the differentiation of the hematopoietic compartment.[11-13,41-45,51,53]

Whatever their molecular and biological functions, a definitive consensus exists concerning the fact that, to cope with DNA cross-links, a cell needs a functional FA pathway. In response to cross-linking agents the FANCA, FANCC, FANCE, FANCF, FANCG and FANCL proteins are assembled in a nuclear complex, named FA core complex or upstream FA complex. The nuclear assembly of the FA core complex is necessary for the activation and focal assembly of both RAD50/MRE11/NBS1 complex and FANCD2.[20,46] Moreover, FA core complex is necessary for the ATR-/ATM-mediated and NBS1-dependent FANCD2 phosphorylation in response to DNA damage.[38,47,50] The FA core complex is not necessary for the activation of FANCD1/BRCA2 and, vice-versa, FANCD1/BRCA2 is not necessary for either FA core complex and FANCD2 activation. Similarly, the functionality of the product of the recently identified FA-J complementation group is not required for FA core complex and FANCD2 activity.[33] Presently, is not known if FANCD1/BRCA2 and the yet uncloned FANCJ participate in the FA pathway defined by the FA core complex, FANCI and FANCD2[6,33,50,59] or if they act independently. It is also unknown if other proteins coassociate with the already known six FANC core complex proteins. Three peptides, namely Fanconi anemia associated proteins (FAAP) of 250, 100 and 90 kDa, were recently isolated in a supramolecular complex which included BLM, RPA, TopoIIIa and the FA core complex.[37] It remains to be determined if FAAP proteins belong to the FA core complex and/or represent new FA genes.

What is known is that the FANC core formation needs the presence of all currently identified participants and also of the product of the gene mutated in FA-B cells.

FANCB

FANCB is one of the uncloned FA genes. FA-B is one of the earlier identified complementation group, although the chromosomal location of *FANCB* remains to be determined. A recently published work reported biallelic inactivation of *BRCA2* as responsible for both FA-B and FA-D1 complementation groups.[25] The link between the germinal homozygous mutations in *BRCA2* and *FANCD1* was validated by the ectopic correction of the MMC hypersensitivity of a FA-D1 cell line and confirmed extensively by the identification of mutations in all known FA-D1 patients. On the contrary, concerning FA-B, mutations in the *BRCA2* gene have not been observed in others patients classified in that group. In light of that, the original mutations identified[25] are probably polymorphisms or hypomorphic variant not linked to the FA phenotype. Although unknown, FANCB is necessary to both FANCA phosphorylation and FANCA/FANCG interaction which seem to be the first steps leading to the nuclear accumulation of the FA core complex.

FANCG

FANCG was cloned by the functional complementation of a FA-G cell line and its involvement in FA syndrome was confirmed by the identification of inactivating mutations in four FA-G cell lines. The sequence appeared to be identical to the previously identified human gene *XRCC9*, which was able to complement the DNA damage hypersensitivity of the XRCC9 cell mutant, derived from the Chinese hamster cell line UV40.[9] The *XRCC9* gene was localized to chromosome band 9p13,[34] a region in which a potential FA gene has been localized using homozygosity mapping.[52] *FANCG/XRCC9* encodes a 2.5-kb mRNA highly expressed in human testis.[34] In human lymphoblasts, mutation in *FANCA, FANCE* and *FANCF* lowered the expression of *FANCG/XRCC9* mRNA.[9] Ectopic expression of the wt *FANCG* cDNA in FA-G cells corrects the MMC hypersensitivity of the cells and increases *FANCA* expression.[18] Reciprocally, in ectopically corrected FA-A cells an increased expression of *FANCG* was noticed. FA-G corrected cells show also an improved expression of *FANCC*.[19]

The translation of the *FANCG/XRCC9* mRNA results in a polypeptide of 622 amino acids,[9,34] showing an apparent molecular weight of 63kDa.[19,61] By using a homology search strategy, the presence of seven tetratricopeptide repeat motifs (TPR) covering FANCG has been identified.[3] These repeats are known to function as scaffolds mediating protein-protein interactions.[23,32] In undamaged wild-type FA pathway cells, the protein is distributed in both cytoplasm and nucleus.

By using yeast 2- and 3-hybrid systems, in vitro pull down, ex-vivo immunoprecipitation or in vivo cytological analysis, it has been established that FANCG directly and strongly interacts with FANCA.[22,26,48] The interaction is critical for the reciprocal increasing in FANCA and FANCG cellular content observed in FA-A or FA-G corrected cells.[19] The FANCG/FANCA interaction extended the half-life of both proteins from 1 to 10 hours. The optimal formation of the FANCG/FANCA complex requires FANCB, FANCC and FANCF but is independent of FANCD1/BRCA2, FANCD2 and FANCE.[60] Moreover, formation of the FANCG/FANCA complex is a prerequisite for FANCC binding to FANCA to form a ternary complex. Importantly, the proper accumulation of FANCG in the nucleus requires also the other components of the complex and FANCB.[19] FANCA/FANCG interaction is required to restore MMC resistance.[29] By using several FANCG mutants, it has been reported that the N- (1-367) and C- (511-622) terminal region of FANCG are involved in FANCA interactions, but that the full length protein is necessary for an optimal interaction. FANCG binds to the N-terminal NLS of FANCA.[26,31] Mutant expressed forms of FANCA bind with FANCG and retain it in the cytoplasm.[18] It has been demonstrated that FANCG interacts also with FANCF.[22] On the contrary, no interaction was observed with FANCC and FANCE.[22,26,48] In the yeast 2-hybrid system, a weak interaction was also observed among FANCG polypeptides encompassing the 1-313 region, suggesting a possible dimerization.[26] Altogether, these observations lead to the proposal that FANCG plays a key role in assembly and/or stabilization of the FA core complex.

Moreover, FANCG interacts with FANCD1/BRCA2 in the yeast 2-hybrid system. Both proteins immunoprecipitate and FANCG colocalizes with MMC-induced BRCA2 foci. Two regions in BRCA2, covering the aminoacids 499-994 and 2350-2545, are involved in the interaction with FANCG.[27]

FANCG seems to play a double connecting role: one as the glue of the FANC core complex and the other possibly linking the complex to BRCA2 activity. However, the role of the FANCG/BRCA2 interaction remains to be established, since BRCA2 and RAD51 are normally recruited to crosslinked DNA in FA-G as well as in the other FA-core complex cell mutants.[21] This suggests that crosslinkers follow two independent pathways to activate the FA core complex and FANCD1/BRCA2, and that, in spite of their colocalization, the activation and focalization of FANCD2 and RAD51 are mutually independent events.

Remembering the potential involvement of FA proteins in other biological pathways than DNA damage responses, it is important to note that FANCG was identified as a phosphoprotein which can be induced and phosphorylated in response to TNF-alpha treatment, a process that appears to be NF-κB dependent.[17]

It has also been shown that FANCG interacts with cytochrome P450 2E1 (CYP2E1).[16] As a member of the P450 super family, CYP2E1 is involved in free radicals production and activation of pro-DNA damaging agents. In FA-G cells, CYP2E1 was over-expressed and over-induced by MMC, whereas its expression was undetectable in ectopically corrected FA-G cells and in normal lymphoblasts.[16] The FANCG/CYP2E1 interaction was independently confirmed by a yeast 2-hybrid screen.[49] During that screen, several other FANCG interactors were isolated, including the transposon derived Buster 1 transposon-like protein, the prosome b subunit, the Placental Lactogen Hormone, a novel SH2 containing protein (NSP2, accession N° AF124250) and a hypothetical protein, believed to be SOCS (accession N° NM_017873).[49] The potential link(s) of those proteins with FA remain to be analyzed.

Similarly to *FANCA* and *FANCC* mutants, *FANCG* mice show normal viability and no major developmental abnormalities, but germ cell defects and decreased fertility. Lymphocytes, bone marrow cells and fibroblasts have spontaneous chromosome fragility and MMC hypersensitivity.[62]

FANCF

FANCF was cloned by functional complementation. The gene was located on chromosome 11p15. The *FANCF* ORF, which is not interrupted by introns, encodes a protein of 374aa with a molecular mass of 42kD. An homology search analysis revealed the presence of a homology region between FANCF and the prokaryotic RNA-binding protein ROM.[8]

By both cellular fractionation and analysis of GFP-tagged FANCF transiently transfected cells, it has been determined that FANCF is predominantly localized in the nucleus. Since its presence in that cell compartment was observed in FA core complex mutated cells, it is likely that the nuclear localization of FANCF is independent of the other FA proteins. FANCF immunoprecipitates in vivo with FANCA, FANCC, FANCE and FANCG. The interaction between these proteins is present in FANCD1/BRCA2 and FANCD2 cells. Lack of FANCF did not alter the cytoplasmic/nuclear partitioning of FANCA. By in vitro pull-down experiments and yeast 2-hybrid analysis, it has been established that only FANCG interact directly with FANCF. Although unable to interact directly with FANCA or FANCC, FANCF stabilizes their interaction.

FANCE

FANCE is localized on chromosome 6p.[61] *FANCE* codes for a nuclear protein of 58kDa with a predicted bipartite nuclear localization signal[7] that promotes the nuclear accumulation of and interacts with FANCC. Mainly located in the cell nucleus, irrespective of the expression of other FA proteins, FANCE coimmunoprecipitates with FANCA, FANCC and FANCG and it is necessary to FANCC nuclear accumulation and for an optimal FANCC expression.[56]

As a component of the FA core complex, FANCE is required for monoubiquitination of FANCD2 and assembly of FANCD2 foci. Moreover, FANCE interacts and colocalizes with FANCD2.[39]

The yeast 2-hybrid system has validated the direct interaction of FANCE with FANCC or FANCD2.[22] Since FANCD2 was never coimmunoprecipitated with FANCC, it may be inferred that the interactions FANCE/FANCC and FANCE/FANCD2 are independent. It will be interesting to know if those interactions are mutually exclusive and sequential.

FA-E cells show a higher basal level of 8-OHdG and a defect in the repair of H_2O_2-induced DNA damage.[63]

Conclusion

In conclusion, during the last number of years significant effort has been exerted to increase our understanding of the FA pathway, nevertheless, precise biological activities and the roles of the FANC proteins remain still undetermined (Fig. 1). The complexity of the biochemical and

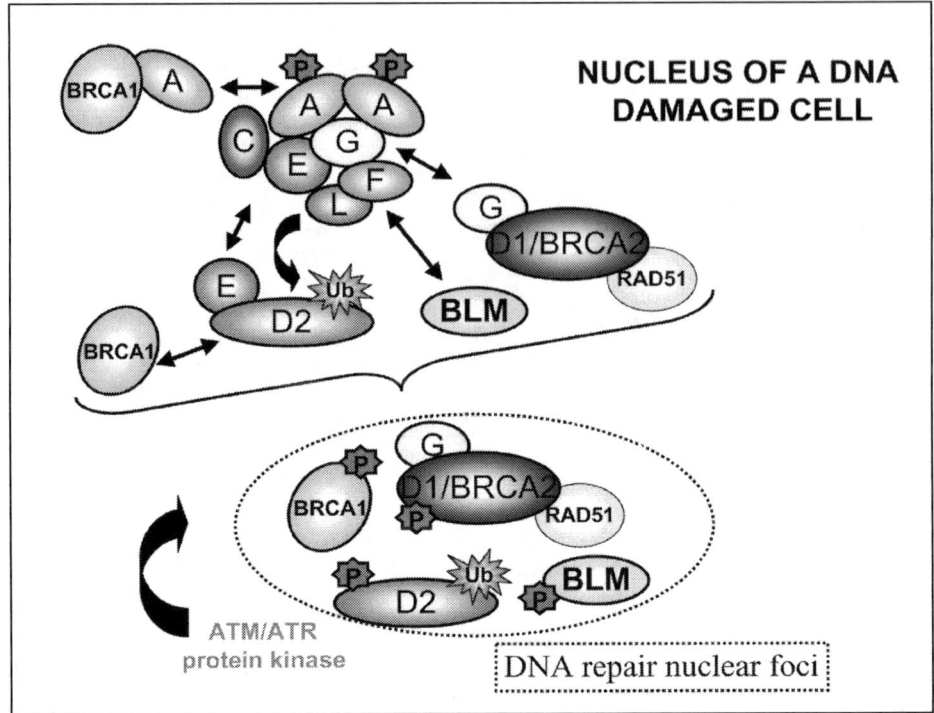

Figure 1. Nuclear activation of the FANC pathway. In response to induced DNA damage the Fanconi anemia core complex is assembled in the cell nucleus leading to the activation of FANCD2 and the formation of DNA-repair nuclear foci. BRCA1, FANCD2, FANCD1/BRCA2 and RAD51 are among the several proteins that participate to foci formation. The proposed model derives from data presented by several reported authors.

functional interactions of the FANC proteins suggests that they may integrate different processes, including but not limited to cell cycle checkpoints, DNA repair and the metabolism of DNA-damaging agents, involved in the control of the genomic stability.

Note Added in Proof

FANCB was recently identified by Meetei and coll. (Nat Genet, doi:10.1038/ng1458). Surprisingly, the gene coding for FANCB was localized at Xp22.31. Consequently, the individuals belonging to FA-B complementation group are male. As expected, FANCB is an essential component of the FA core complex required for FANCD2 monoubiquination.

References

1. Ahmad SI, Hanaoka F, Kirk SH. Molecular biology of Fanconi anaemia—an old problem, a new insight. Bioessays 2002; 24:439-48.
2. Alter BP. Cancer in Fanconi anemia 1927-2001. Cancer 2003; 97:425-40.
3. Blom E, van de Vrugt HJ, de Vries Y et al. Multiple TPR motifs characterize the Fanconi anemia FANCG protein. DNA Repair (Amst) 2004; 3:77-84.
4. Buchwald M, Moustacchi E. Is Fanconi anemia caused by a defect in the processing of DNA damage? Mutat Res 1998; 408:75-90.
5. Cumming RC, Lightfoot J, Beard K et al. Fanconi anemia group C protein prevents apoptosis in hematopoietic cells through redox regulation of GSTP1. Nat Med 2001; 7:814-20.
6. D'Andrea AD, Grompe M. The Fanconi anaemia/BRCA pathway. Nat Rev Cancer. 2003; 3:23-34.
7. de Winter JP, Leveille F, van Berkel CG et al. Isolation of a cDNA representing the Fanconi anemia complementation group E gene. Am J Hum Genet 2000a; 67:1306-8.

8. de Winter JP, Rooimans MA, van Der Weel L et al The Fanconi anaemia gene FANCF encodes a novel protein with homology to ROM. Nat Genet 2000b; 24:15-6.
9. de Winter JP, Waisfisz Q, Rooimans MA et al. The Fanconi anaemia group G gene FANCG is identical with XRCC9. Nat Genet 1998; 20:281-3.
10. Duckworth-Rysiecki G, Cornish K, Clarke CA et al. Identification of two complementation groups in Fanconi anemia. Somat Cell Mol Genet 1985; 11:35-41.
11. Dufour C, Corcione A, Svahn J et al. TNF-alpha and IFN-gamma are overexpressed in the bone marrow of Fanconi anemia patients and TNF-alpha suppresses erythropoiesis in vitro. Blood 2003; 102:2053-9, (Epub 2003 May 15).
12. Fagerlie S, Lensch MW, Pang Q et al. The Fanconi anemia group C gene product: Signaling functions in hematopoietic cells. Exp Hematol 2001a; 29:1371-81.
13. Fagerlie SR, Diaz J, Christianson TA et al. Functional correction of FA-C cells with FANCC suppresses the expression of interferon gamma-inducible genes. Blood 2001b; 97:3017-24.
14. Faivre L, Guardiola P, Lewis C et.al. Association of complementation group and mutation type with clinical outcome in fanconi anemia. European Fanconi Anemia Research Group. Blood 2000; 96:4064-70.
15. Fanconi anaemia/breast cancer consortium. Positional cloning of the Fanconi anaemia group A gene. The Nat Genet 1996; 14:324-8.
16. Futaki M, Igarashi T, Watanabe S et al. The FANCG Fanconi anemia protein interacts with CYP2E1: Possible role in protection against oxidative DNA damage. Carcinogenesis 2002; 23:67-72.
17. Futaki M, Watanabe S, Kajigaya S et al. Fanconi anemia protein, FANCG, is a phosphoprotein and is upregulated with FANCA after TNF-alpha treatment. Biochem Biophys Res Commun 2001; 281:347-51.
18. Garcia-Higuera I, Kuang Y, Denham J et al. The fanconi anemia proteins FANCA and FANCG stabilize each other and promote the nuclear accumulation of the Fanconi anemia complex. Blood 2000; 96:3224-30.
19. Garcia-Higuera I, Kuang Y, Naf D et al. Fanconi anemia proteins FANCA, FANCC, and FANCG/XRCC9 interact in a functional nuclear complex. Mol Cell Biol 1999; 19:4866-73.
20. Garcia-Higuera I, Taniguchi T, Ganesan S et al. Interaction of the Fanconi anemia proteins and BRCA1 in a common pathway. Mol Cell 2001; 7:249-62.
21. Godthelp BC, Artwert F, Joenje H et al. Impaired DNA damage-induced nuclear Rad51 foci formation uniquely characterizes Fanconi anemia group D1. Oncogene 2002; 21:5002-5.
22. Gordon SM, Buchwald M. Fanconi anemia protein complex: Mapping protein interactions in the yeast 2- and 3-hybrid systems. Blood 2003; 102:136-41.
23. Groves MR, Barford D. Topological characteristics of helical repeat proteins. Curr Opin Struct Biol 1999; 9:383-9.
24. Hoshino T, Wang J, Devetten MP et al. Molecular chaperone GRP94 binds to the Fanconi anemia group C protein and regulates its intracellular expression. Blood 1998; 91:4379-86.
25. Howlett NG, Taniguchi T, Olson S et al. Biallelic inactivation of BRCA2 in Fanconi anemia. Science 2002; 297:606-9.
26. Huber PA, Medhurst AL, Youssoufian H et al. Investigation of Fanconi anemia protein interactions by yeast two-hybrid analysis. Biochem Biophys Res Commun 2000; 268:73-7.
27. Hussain S, Witt E, Huber PA et al. Direct interaction of the Fanconi anemia protein FANCG with BRCA2/FANCD1. Hum Mol Genet 2003; 5:5.
28. Joenje H, Oostra AB, Wijker M et al. Evidence for at least eight Fanconi anemia genes. Am J Hum Genet 1997; 61:940-4.
29. Kruyt FA, Abou-Zahr F, Mok H et al. Resistance to mitomycin C requires direct interaction between the Fanconi anemia proteins FANCA and FANCG in the nucleus through an arginine-rich domain. J Biol Chem 1999; 274:34212-8.
30. Kruyt FA, Hoshino T, Liu JM et al. Abnormal microsomal detoxification implicated in Fanconi anemia group C by interaction of the FAC protein with NADPH cytochrome P450 reductase. Blood 1998; 92:3050-6.
31. Kuang Y, Garcia-Higuera I, Moran A et al. Carboxy terminal region of the Fanconi anemia protein FANCG/XRCC9 is required for functional activity. Blood 2000; 96:1625-32.
32. Lamb JR, Tugendreich S, Hieter P. Tetratrico peptide repeat interactions: To TPR or not to TPR? Trends Biochem Sci 1995; 20:257-9.
33. Levitus M, Rooimans MA, Steltenpool J et al. Heterogeneity in Fanconi anemia: Evidence for 2 new genetic subtypes. Blood 2004; 103:2498-503, (Epub 2003).
34. Liu N, Lamerdin JE, Tucker JD et al. The human XRCC9 gene corrects chromosomal instability and mutagen sensitivities in CHO UV40 cells. Proc Natl Acad Sci USA 1997; 94:9232-7.
35. Lo Ten Foe JR, Rooimans MA, Bosnoyan-Collins L et al. Expression cloning of a cDNA for the major Fanconi anaemia gene FAA. Nat Genet 1996; 14:320-3.

36. Meetei AR, de Winter JP, Medhurst AL et al. A novel ubiquitin ligase is deficient in Fanconi anemia. Nat Genet 2003a; 35:165-70, (Epub 2003 Sep 14).
37. Meetei AR, Sechi S, Wallisch M et al. A multiprotein nuclear complex connects Fanconi anemia and Bloom syndrome. Mol Cell Biol 2003b; 23:3417-26.
38. Nakanishi K, Taniguchi T, Ranganathan V et al. Interaction of FANCD2 and NBS1 in the DNA damage response. Nat Cell Biol 2002; 4:913-20.
39. Pace P, Johnson M, Tan WM et al. FANCE: The link between Fanconi anaemia complex assembly and activity. EMBO J 2002; 21:3414-23.
40. Pagano G, Youssoufian H. Fanconi anaemia proteins: Major roles in cell protection against oxidative damage. Bioessays 2003; 25:589-95.
41. Pang Q, Christianson TA, Keeble W et al. The anti-apoptotic function of Hsp70 in the interferon-inducible double-stranded RNA-dependent protein kinase-mediated death signaling pathway requires the Fanconi anemia protein, FANCC. J Biol Chem 2002; 277:49638-43, (Epub 2002 Oct 22).
42. Pang Q, Christianson TA, Koretsky T et al. Nucleophosmin interacts with and inhibits the catalytic function of eukaryotic initiation factor 2 kinase PKR. J Biol Chem 2003; 278:41709-17, (Epub 2003 Jul 25).
43. Pang Q, Fagerlie S, Christianson TA et al. The Fanconi anemia protein FANCC binds to and facilitates the activation of STAT1 by gamma interferon and hematopoietic growth factors. Mol Cell Biol 2000; 20:4724-35.
44. Pang Q, Keeble W, Christianson TA et al. FANCC interacts with Hsp70 to protect hematopoietic cells from IFN-gamma/TNF-alpha-mediated cytotoxicity. EMBO J 2001a; 20:4478-89.
45. Pang Q, Keeble W, Diaz J et al. Role of double-stranded RNA-dependent protein kinase in mediating hypersensitivity of Fanconi anemia complementation group C cells to interferon gamma, tumor necrosis factor-alpha, and double-stranded RNA. Blood 2001b; 97:1644-52.
46. Pichierri P, Averbeck D, Rosselli F. DNA cross-link-dependent RAD50/MRE11/NBS1 subnuclear assembly requires the Fanconi anemia C protein. Hum Mol Genet 2002; 11:2531-46.
47. Pichierri P, Rosselli F. The DNA crosslink-induced S-phase checkpoint depends on ATR-CHK1 and ATR-NBS1-FANCD2 pathways. EMBO J 2004; 26:26.
48. Reuter T, Herterich S, Bernhard O et al. Strong FANCA/FANCG but weak FANCA/FANCC interaction in the yeast 2-hybrid system. Blood 2000; 95:719-20.
49. Reuter TY, Medhurst AL, Waisfisz Q et al. Yeast two-hybrid screens imply involvement of Fanconi anemia proteins in transcription regulation, cell signaling, oxidative metabolism, and cellular transport. Exp Cell Res 2003; 289:211-21.
50. Rosselli F, Briot D, Pichierri P. The Fanconi anemia pathway and the DNA interstrand cross-links repair. Biochimie 2003; 85:1175-84.
51. Rosselli F, Sanceau J, Gluckman E et al. Abnormal lymphokine production: A novel feature of the genetic disease Fanconi anemia. II. In vitro and in vivo spontaneous overproduction of tumor necrosis factor alpha. Blood 1994; 83:1216-25.
52. Saar K, Schindler D, Wegner RD et al. Localisation of a Fanconi anaemia gene to chromosome 9p. Eur J Hum Genet 1998; 6:501-8.
53. Schultz JC, Shahidi NT. Tumor necrosis factor-alpha overproduction in Fanconi's anemia. Am J Hematol 1993; 42:196-201.
54. Strathdee CA, Duncan AM, Buchwald M. Evidence for at least four Fanconi anaemia genes including FACC on chromosome 9. Nat Genet 1992a; 1:196-8.
55. Strathdee CA, Gavish H, Shannon WR et al. Cloning of cDNAs for Fanconi's anaemia by functional complementation. Nature 1992b; 358:434.
56. Taniguchi T, D'Andrea AD. The Fanconi anemia protein, FANCE, promotes the nuclear accumulation of FANCC. Blood 2002; 100:2457-62.
57. Timmers C, Taniguchi T, Hejna J et al. Positional cloning of a novel Fanconi anemia gene FANCD2. Mol Cell 2001; 7:241-8.
58. Tischkowitz MD, Hodgson SV. Fanconi anaemia. J Med Genet 2003; 40:1-10.
59. Venkitaraman AR. Tracing the network connecting brca and fanconi anaemia proteins. Nat Rev Cancer 2004; 4:266-76.
60. Waisfisz Q, de Winter JP, Kruyt FA et al. A physical complex of the Fanconi anemia proteins FANCG/XRCC9 and FANCA. Proc Natl Acad Sci USA 1999a; 96:10320-5.
61. Waisfisz Q, Saar K, Morgan NV et al. The Fanconi anemia group E gene FANCE maps to chromosome 6p. Am J Hum Genet 1999b; 64:1400-5.
62. Yang Y, Kuang Y, De Oca RM et al. Targeted disruption of the murine Fanconi anemia gene Fancg/Xrcc9. Blood 2001; 98:3435-40.
63. Zunino A, Degan P, Vigo T et al. Hydrogen peroxide: Effects on DNA chromosomes cell cycle and apoptosis induction in Fanconi's anemia cell lines. Mutagenesis 2001; 16:283-8.

CHAPTER 6

FANCD1/BRCA2 and FANCD2

Gary M. Kupfer*

The field of FA was both excited as well as surprised when the first cloned genes encoded proteins that resembled no known protein motif. Several binding proteins were described, yet no biochemical function could be discerned. Now, 11 years after the cloning of FANCC, we have in hand 12 *FA* genes, and the FA field has turned 180° from one dealing with orphan proteins to one well-ensconced in the mainstream of cancer biology: the FANCD1 and FANCD2 proteins are BRCA2 and a BRCA1 interactor, respectively. We now have the ability to assess FA function in the context of the biochemistry of these proteins, which are the subject of intense focus. In addition, we now have a potential mechanism for the modification of FANCD2: FANCL, the latest *FA* gene to be cloned, may be the ubiquitin ligase responsible for the monoubiquitination of FANCD2. This would represent the first biochemical mechanism established in the FA pathway response to DNA damage.

The FA-D Complementation Group

At the time of the cloning of the first *FA* gene, FANCC, it was also apparent that more complementation groups existed for FA, based on somatic cell hybridization experiments.[1,2] A reference cell line for FA-D was first reported in 1992. The first major biochemical advance in FA was made in the description of the FANCA-FANCC interaction, an interaction dependent upon a wild-type genetic background.[3] What became apparent, however, was that the FA-D complementation group was different: FANCA, FANCC, and FANCG formed a complex in mutant FA-D cells, indicating unique properties of this complementation group.[4]

Genes and Their Proteins Products

FANCD2

After delineation of FA-D reference cell line, microcell fusions using minichromosomes revealed that the FA-D locus was 3p22-26.[5] Eventually, the Grompe group worked their way through expressed sequence tags and cloning of a candidate *FANCD* gene.[6,7] Testing of the putative gene clarified the FA-D complementation group. Mutations were only found in a subset of proposed FA-D cell lines, namely PD20 (Table 1).[7] Once expression of FANCD was modulated, it clearly only corrected the PD20 cell line and not other FA-D reference cell lines, such as HSC62. FANCD2 was in fact absent in PD20 cells. Hence, the nomenclature was changed to reflect this outcome, and the newly cloned gene was termed FANCD2.

FANCD2 is a 4356 base pair cDNA with 44 exons. The gene is found in databases of higher eukaryotes including mouse, *Drosophila*, *Arabidopsis*, and *C. elegans*. No yeast homolog has been identified.[8]

---

*Gary M. Kupfer—Department of Microbiology and Department of Pediatrics, Division of Pediatric Hematology-Oncology University of Virginia, Charlottesville, Virginia 22903, U.S.A. Email: gk9e@virginia.edu

Molecular Mechanisms of Fanconi Anemia, edited by Shamim I. Ahmad and Sandra H. Kirk. ©2006 Eurekah.com and Springer Science+Business Media.

The protein sequence reveals a predicted protein of 150 kD with the only discernible motifs consisting of nuclear localization signal and high mobility group domains. Immunoblotting reveals a consistent 150 kD protein band with a variably expressed higher mobility form. This form, pegged the "FANCD2-L (long)" is most highly expressed after DNA damage and during S phase. The FA core complex, composed of FANCA, FANCC, FANCE, FANCF, FANCG, and FANCL, appears to be required for FANCD2-L to form, as FANCD2-L is absent in all the FA core complex complementation groups. However, the core complex, which forms in FA-D1 and FA-D2, is not sufficient for FANCD2-L, since FANCD2-L is not present in FA-I cells, a group which contains both the core complex and FANCD2. The FANCD2-L is not a universal marker for FA, as it forms in FA-D1 and FA-J cells; nonetheless, the vast majority of FA patients fall within the groups in which FANCD2-L is absent.[7,9,10]

FANCD2 was analyzed by mass spectroscopy, and ubiquitination was detected at lysine 561.[10] Mutation of this lysine and subsequent FANCD2 expression revealed the functional importance of the lysine, as FANCD2(K561A) was incapable of correcting the mitomycin C (MMC) hypersensitivity of FA-D2 cells. As FA core complex formation has been shown to be abolished in most complementation groups, ubiquitinated FANCD2 is abrogated in all complementation groups except FA-D1 and FA-J, also indicating its functional importance. The detection of this form of FANCD2 and its absence in mutant FA cells has been proposed as a new tool in the diagnostics of FA.[9,11]

FANCD2 localizes to the nucleus. In a similar manner as the immunoblotting experiments, immunofluorescence revealed that endogenous FANCD2 localized to nuclear foci in a DNA damage and S phase inducible manner.[10] Curiously, these dots have been shown to colocalize with BRCA1 and RAD51 foci,[12] and coprecipitation experiments by the D'Andrea group have confirmed the physical interaction of BRCA1 and FANCD2.[10] Further studies have also joined FANCD2 and NBS1 in colocalizing foci after DNA damage.[13]

The relatedness of BRCA1 to the biochemical story of FA is a logical one in light of the DNA damage hypersensitivity of the BRCA1 mutant cells. However, in spite of this association, no increase in breast cancer susceptibility has been reported in FA patients or in heterozygote relatives of probands, except in a recent analysis that looked at FA kindreds with BRCA2 mutations.[18] The relative lack of patients historically surviving to adulthood and the rarity of FA generally make an epidemiological study difficult, although this may be countered by more surviving FA patients due to more successful stem cell transplantation. What may be more demonstrable is the connection of aberrant FA protein expression in cancers in the nonFA population, such as ovarian, head and neck, and myeloid leukemia, as has recently been reported.[19-21]

BRCA1 -/- cells, however, are hypersensitive to DNA damage, including MMC and IR.[22,23] Thus, the question of ionizing radiation sensitivity comes up at this point. FA cells have shown some measure of modest radiation sensitivity, although not consistently.[24-27] For example, conditioning for FA patients must be dose reduced when receiving radiation for stem cell transplantation.[28] Also, some investigators have demonstrated differential sensitivity to IR in FA mutant cells in the form of increased cytotoxicity and chromosomal breakage and sensitivity to radiomimetic agents. Contrastingly, this has not been universally true amongst all complementation groups. For example, mouse knockout cells are variably sensitive to radiation, and the observed sensitivity in human mutant FA cells is not as great as in ataxia telangiectasia mutant cells nor is it as much as that induced by MMC.[25,29,30]

BRCA1, through a complex with its partner BARD1, also has E3 ubiquitin ligase activity, leading to the suggestion that BRCA1 could be the enzyme whereby FANCD2 is ubiquitinated.[31,32] A report by Moses' group suggests decreased ubiquitination of FANCD2 in BRCA1 RNAi knockdown cells.[33] This hypothesis has been countered by 2 recent reports. First, Patel's group showed that monoubiquitination of FANCD2 was independent of BRCA1 in BRCA1 RNAi knockdown cells.[34] Second, a newly cloned FA gene, FANCL, exhibits E3 ligase activity in vitro.[14]

What remains clear is that the monoubiquitination of FANCD2 is a central hallmark of wild-type FA function in almost every complementation group, except rare groups such as FA-D1 and FA-J.[7,9,10] Thus, this modification depends upon wild-type FA core complex (FANCA, FANCC, FANCE, FANCF, FANCG, FANCL). A physical connection between FANCD2 and the core complex has been established as well. Patel's group described FANCE-FANCD2 interaction through coprecipitation and colocalization.[17] In addition, Gordon and Buchwald have reported 2 hybrid data that define the binding domain with FANCE to the N terminus of FANCD2.[35] Others have reported further connections with the FA core complex. Moses' group showed by 2 hybrid and coprecipitation an interaction between FANCA and BRCA1.[36]

Since BRCA1 exists in a large macromolecular complex approaching 2 MD, the other members of this complex, termed BASC for BRCA1 associated supercomplex, become potential partners for FANCD2 as well.[37] Because of the possible link to IR sensitivity and the existence of another DNA damage hypersensitivity syndrome, ataxia telangiectasia, D'Andrea's group assessed the importance of the ATM kinase in FANCD2.[25] ATM is a coprecipitating protein in the BASC complex and phosphorylates BRCA1. The D'Andrea group detected a phosphorylation of FANCD2 at serine 222 by ATM. Curiously, while abolishing IR resistance, the mutation of FANCD2 at serine 222 did not abolish the ability to correct MMC sensitivity in FA-D2 cells. These data indicate that the FANCD2 protein may be multifunctional or serve as a junction point for cross talk between 2 different pathways (ATM and FA) that respond to distinct types of DNA damage. In sum, the findings of interaction of FANCD2 in some manner with BRCA1, RAD51, and ATM hint strongly that FA biochemistry may play a direct or indirect role in homologous recombination (HR), a process likely to play a role in resolution of DNA cross links.[12,13] Defective RAD51 foci formation has been noted to be in some way deficient in FA cells in general[38] or specifically only to FA-D1 cells.[39] These connections have been made in a variety of ways in cell biology studies. Takata and colleagues measured a reduced rate of HR in FA cells,[40] while increased activity was demonstrated by Campbell's group.[41]

Recently, Grompe and workers have reported a fascinating knockout mouse for FANCD2 that may prove more informative than previous knockout mice knocked out for *FA* genes, which yielded cancer-free phenotypes. In contrast, the fancd2 knockout displays epithelial cancer and an intact ATM pathway and is similar in many ways to the BRCA2 hypomorphs.[42]

FANCD1/BRCA2

Because of the connection with BRCA1, it was a logical extension to consider BRCA2 as a potential *FA* gene. Sequencing of BRCA2 was conducted on the "other" FA-D cell lines, now termed FA-D1, in which the FA core complex forms. Given the enormity of the *BRCA2* gene, this task proved to be weighty. Identified mutations were proved to be functionally important as transduction back into FA-D1 cells failed to correct for MMC hypersensitivity while wild-type BRCA2 did indeed correct (Table 1).[43] This analysis was extended to other FA lines, including FA-B cells. In these cells, putative BRCA2 mutations were identified, but a clear correction of MMC sensitivity was not possible since these cells are not markedly sensitive or easily transducible in the first place. Thus the identification of FA-B as FA-D1/BRCA2 remains circumstantial.

Mutations in BRCA2, as BRCA1, lead to predisposition to breast and ovarian cancer in a classic two hit fashion.[44,45] BRCA2 is a 380 kD protein with multiple RAD51 binding domains, an N terminal transactivation domain, and a single stranded DNA binding domain at the C terminus.[46] As in BRCA1, the BRCA2-null knockout mice are embryonic lethal,[47] implying that FA patients in the FA-D1 group have some partially functional BRCA2. Null BRCA2 and BRCA1 cells are MMC-sensitive, and partially disrupted BRCA2 mice, which preserves the N terminus of BRCA2, results in a phenotype similar to FA.[48-52]

As in BRCA1 mutations, BRCA2 mutations appear to be associated with a near 80% risk of breast cancer, as well as heightened risk for ovarian, pancreatic, gastric, and colon cancer.[46] As

Table 1. FANCD1/BRCA2 and FANCD2 mutations

FANCD2 mutations (from Timmers, 2001(7))	
PD20	S126G/splice
	R1263H
VU008	R302W
	Q320X
PD733	exon 17 deletion (homozygous)
FANCD1/BRCA2	(from Howlett, 2002(43))
HSC62	IVS19-1 G to A exon 20 (homozygous)
EUFA423	7691/insAT exon 15
	9900/insA exon 27
HSC230	3033/del exon 11
	10204 A to T exon 27
EUFA579	7235 G to A exon 13
	5837 TC to AG exon 11
AP37P	8415 G to T exon 18
	8732 C to A exon 20

mentioned earlier, FA-D1 kindreds show increased risk of breast cancer, consistent with having BRCA2 mutations.[18]

Work on BRCA2 has established a new connection with the FA core complex in the 2 hybrid data by Mathew, et.al., showing an interaction between FANCG and BRCA2.[53] On the other hand, Moses' group demonstrated that knockdown of BRCA2 resulted in preservation of FANCD2 ubiquitination, suggesting that BRCA2 is not needed for the execution of FANCD2 monoubiquitination.[33] This is consistent with published reports that FA-D1 cells exhibit monoubiquitination of FANCD2.[54]

Conclusions

Given that the whole of FA biology has now turned its focus on BRCA1/2, the connections to be made across the spectrum of general caretakers of genomic stability are expanding. BRCA1 has been recently characterized at the nexus of the DNA damage response. As mentioned, purification of the BRCA1 complex, termed the BASC complex, has revealed the colocalization of numerous DNA repair proteins, including mismatch repair, BLM, ATM, replication proteins, and the mismatch repair proteins.[37] The RPA, BLM, and ATM are notable in their interaction with the FA proteins, and a recent publication notes the coprecipitation of BLM with FANCA in a low salt extract.[55] For example, as discussed, ATM appears to phosphorylate FANCD2.[25] In addition, BLM and RPA 14/32/70 have all been shown to bind to the FA core complex in a low salt nuclear extract. Unlike BRCA1 knockout cells, BLM mutant cells have not been shown to be crosslinker hypersensitive, so the functional significance of this association is not clear.

All of these data place the FA proteins, including FANCD2 and FANCD1/BRCA2, at the nexus of the DNA damage response in the cell. Nonetheless, the primary biochemical function for these proteins remains unknown, which is clearly the most important area of effort. More questions remain. For example:

- With what other proteins does FANCD2 truly interact and not simply exist together in nuclear foci? How meaningful are nuclear foci?
- Does a FANCD2 complex contain binding proteins encoded by new FA complementation group genes?
- How large is the FANCD2 complex?
- What associated biochemical activities copurify with FANCD2?
- What subcellular compartments contain FANCD2?

Future directions will be achieved biochemically once it is clear what the function of associated proteins might be. Even though the *2 FANCD* genes together stand out as distinctive from the other FA complementation group genes, they nonetheless are inextricably linked by virtue of their functional connection to the FA core complex.

References

1. Strathdee CA, Duncan AMV, Buchwald M. Evidence for at least four Fanconi Anemia genes including FACC on chromosome 9. Nat Genet 1992; 1:196-198.
2. Strathdee CA, Gavish H, Shannon WR et al. Cloning of cDNAs for Fanconi's anaemia by functional complementation. Nature 1992; 356:763-767.
3. Kupfer GM, Naf D, Suliman A et al. The Fanconi anaemia proteins, FAA and FAC, interact to form a nuclear complex. Nat Genet 1997; 17:487-490.
4. Yamashita T, Kupfer G, Naf D et al. The Fanconi Anemia Pathway Requires FAA Phosphorylation and FAA/FAC Nuclear Accumulation. PNAS 1998; 95:13085-13090.
5. Whitney M et al. Microcell mediated chromosome transfer maps the Fanconi anemia group D gene to chromosome 3p. Nature Genet 1995; 11:341-343.
6. Hejna JA, Timmers CD, Reifsteck C et al. Localization of the Fanconi anemia complementation group D gene to a 200-kb region on chromosome 3p25.3. Am J Hum Genet 2000; 66:1540-1551.
7. Timmers C, Taniguchi T, Hejna J et al. Positional cloning of a novel Fanconi anemia gene, FANCD2. Mol Cell 2001; 7:241-248.
8. Joenje H, Patel KJ. The emerging genetic and molecular basis of Fanconi anaemia. Nat Rev Genet 2001; 2:446-457.
9. Levitus M, Rooimans MA, Steltenpool J et al. Heterogeneity in Fanconi anemia: Evidence for two new genetic subtypes. Blood 2003.
10. Garcia-Higuera I, Taniguchi T, Ganesan S et al. Interaction of the Fanconi anemia proteins and BRCA1 in a common pathway. Mol Cell 2001; 7:249-262.
11. Shimamura A, de Oca RM, Svenson JL et al. A novel diagnostic screen for defects in the Fanconi anemia pathway. Blood 2002; 100:4649-4654.
12. Taniguchi T, Garcia-Higuera I, Andreassen PR et al. S-phase-specific interaction of the Fanconi anemia protein, FANCD2, with BRCA1 and RAD51. Blood 2002; 100:2414-2420.
13. Nakanishi K, Taniguchi T, Ranganathan V et al. Interaction of FANCD2 and NBS1 in the DNA damage response. Nat Cell Biol 2002; 4:913-920.
14. Offit K, Levran O, Mullaney B et al. Shared genetic susceptibility to breast cancer, brain tumors, and Fanconi anemia. J Natl Cancer Inst 2003; 95:1548-1551.
15. Tischkowitz M, Ameziane N, Waisfisz Q et al. Bi-allelic silencing of the Fanconi anaemia gene FANCF in acute myeloid leukaemia. Br J Haematol 2003; 123:469-471.
16. Marsit CJ, Liu M, Nelson HH et al. Inactivation of the Fanconi anemia/BRCA pathway in lung and oral cancers: implications for treatment and survival. Oncogene 2003.
17. Taniguchi T, Tischkowitz M, Ameziane N et al. Disruption of the Fanconi anemia-BRCA pathway in cisplatin-sensitive ovarian tumors. Nat Med 2003; 9:568-574.
18. Tomlinson GE, Chen TT, Stastny VA et al. Characterization of a breast cancer cell line derived from a germ-line BRCA1 mutation carrier. Cancer Res 1998; 58:3237-3242.
19. Scully R, Chen J, Ochs RL et al. Dynamic changes of BRCA1 subnuclear location and phosphorylation state are initiated by DNA damage. Cell 1997; 90:425-435.
20. Kupfer GM, D'Andrea AD. The effect of the Fanconi anemia polypeptide, FAC, upon p53 induction and G2 checkpoint regulation. Blood 1996; 88:1019-1025.
21. Taniguchi T, Garcia-Higuera I, Xu B et al. Convergence of the fanconi anemia and ataxia telangiectasia signaling pathways. Cell 2002; 109:459-472.
22. Alter BP, Young NS. The bone marrow failure syndromes. In: Nathan DG, Oski FA, eds. Hematology of Infancy and Childhood. Vol. 1. Philadelphia: W.B. Saunders, 1993:216-316.
23. Auerbach A, Buchwald M, Joenje H. Fanconi anemia. In: Vogelstein B, Kinzler K, eds. Genetics of Cancer. New York: McGraw-Hill, 1997:317-332.
24. Guardiola P, Socie G, Pasquini R et al. Allogeneic stem cell transplantation for Fanconi anaemia. Severe Aplastic Anaemia Working Party of the EBMT and EUFAR. European Group for Blood and Marrow Transplantation. Bone Marrow Transplant 1998; 21 Suppl 2:S24-27.
25. Koomen M, Cheng NC, van de Vrugt HJ et al. Reduced fertility and hypersensitivity to mitomycin C characterize Fancg/Xrcc9 null mice. Hum Mol Genet 2002; 11:273-281.
26. Yang Y, Kuang Y, De Oca RM et al. Targeted disruption of the murine Fanconi anemia gene, Fancg/Xrcc9. Blood 2001; 98:3435-3440.
27. Joazeiro CA, Weissman AM. RING finger proteins: Mediators of ubiquitin ligase activity. Cell 2000; 102:549-552.

28. Lorick KL, Jensen JP, Fang S et al. RING fingers mediate ubiquitin-conjugating enzyme (E2)-dependent ubiquitination. Proc Natl Acad Sci USA 1999; 96:11364-11369.
29. Bruun D, Folias A, Akkari Y et al. siRNA depletion of BRCA1, but not BRCA2, causes increased genome instability in Fanconi anemia cells. DNA Repair (Amst) 2003; 2:1007-1013.
30. Vandenberg CJ, Gergely F, Ong CY et al. BRCA1-independent ubiquitination of FANCD2. Mol Cell 2003; 12:247-254.
31. Meetei AR, de Winter JP, Medhurst AL, et al. A novel ubiquitin ligase is deficient in Fanconi anemia. Nat Genet 2003;35:165-170.
32. Pace P, Johnson M, Tan WM, et al. FANCE: the link between Fanconi anaemia complex assembly and activity. Embo J 2002; 21:3414-3423.
33. Gordon SM, Buchwald M. Fanconi anemia protein complex: Mapping protein interactions in the yeast 2- and 3-hybrid systems. Blood 2003; 102:136-141.
34. Folias A, Matkovic M, Bruun D et al. BRCA1 interacts directly with the Fanconi anemia protein FANCA. Hum Mol Genet 2002; 11:2591-2597.
35. Wang Y, Cortez D, Yazdi P et al. BASC, a super complex of BRCA1-associated proteins involved in the recognition and repair of aberrant DNA structures. Genes Dev 2000; 14:927-939.
36. Digweed M, Rothe S, Demuth I et al. Attenuation of the formation of DNA-repair foci containing RAD51 in Fanconi anaemia. Carcinogenesis 2002; 23:1121-1126.
37. Godthelp BC, Artwert F, Joenje H et al. Impaired DNA damage-induced nuclear Rad51 foci formation uniquely characterizes Fanconi anemia group D1. Oncogene 2002; 21:5002-5005.
38. Yamamoto K, Ishiai M, Matsushita N et al. Fanconi anemia FANCG protein in mitigating radiation- and enzyme-induced DNA double-strand breaks by homologous recombination in vertebrate cells. Mol Cell Biol 2003; 23:5421-5430.
39. Donahue SL, Lundberg R, Saplis RC et al. Deficient regulation of DNA double-strand break repair in Fanconi anemia fibroblasts. J Biol Chem 2003; 278:29487-29495.
40. Houghtaling S, Timmers C, Noll M et al. Epithelial cancer in Fanconi anemia complementation group D2 (Fancd2) knockout mice. Genes Dev 2003; 17:2021-2035.
41. Howlett NG, Taniguchi T, Olson S et al. Biallelic inactivation of BRCA2 in Fanconi anemia. Science 2002; 297:606-609.
42. Collins N, McManus R, Wooster R et al. Consistent loss of the wild type allele in breast cancers from a family linked to the BRCA2 gene on chromosome 13q12-13. Oncogene 1995; 10:1673-1675.
43. Gudmundsson J, Johannesdottir G, Bergthorsson JT et al. Different tumor types from BRCA2 carriers show wild-type chromosome deletions on 13q12-q13. Cancer Res 1995; 55:4830-4832.
44. Powell SN, Kachnic LA. Roles of BRCA1 and BRCA2 in homologous recombination, DNA replication fidelity and the cellular response to ionizing radiation. Oncogene 2003; 22:5784-5791.
45. Hakem R, de la Pompa JL, Mak TW. Developmental studies of Brca1 and Brca2 knock-out mice. J Mammary Gland Biol Neoplasia 1998; 3:431-445.
46. Patel KJ, Yu VP, Lee H et al. Involvement of Brca2 in DNA repair. Mol Cell 1998; 1:347-357.
47. Tutt A, Gabriel A, Bertwistle D et al. Absence of Brca2 causes genome instability by chromosome breakage and loss associated with centrosome amplification. Curr Biol 1999; 9:1107-1110.
48. Moynahan ME, Cui TY, Jasin M. Homology-directed dna repair, mitomycin-c resistance, and chromosome stability is restored with correction of a Brca1 mutation. Cancer Res 2001; 61:4842-4850.
49. Connor F, Bertwistle D, Mee PJ et al. Tumorigenesis and a DNA repair defect in mice with a truncating Brca2 mutation. Nat Genet 1997; 17:423-430.
50. McAllister KA, Bennett LM, Houle CD et al. Cancer susceptibility of mice with a homozygous deletion in the COOH-terminal domain of the Brca2 gene. Cancer Res 2002; 62:990-994.
51. Hussain S, Witt E, Huber PA et al. Direct interaction of the Fanconi anaemia protein FANCG with BRCA2/FANCD1. Hum Mol Genet 2003.
52. Siddique MA, Nakanishi K, Taniguchi T et al. Function of the Fanconi anemia pathway in Fanconi anemia complementation group F and D1 cells. Exp Hematol 2001; 29:1448-1455.
53. Meetei AR, Sechi S, Wallisch M et al. A multiprotein nuclear complex connects Fanconi anemia and Bloom syndrome. Mol Cell Biol 2003; 23:3417-3426.

CHAPTER 7

The *FANC* Genome Surveillance Complex

Takayuki Yamashita*

Historical Overview

FA is an autosomal recessive genetic disorder characterized by progressive bone marrow failure, congenital anomalies and susceptibility to hematological and solid malignancies. The most consistent feature of FA cells is their hypersensitivity to DNA cross-linking agents such as diepoxybutane (DEB) and mitomycin C (MMC). These chemicals at low concentrations induce higher levels of chromosome breakage and cell death in FA cell lines than in control cells. Genetic heterogeneity of FA was shown by complementation analyses based on the cellular hypersensitivity to DNA cross-linking agents (see Chapter 3). Since initial identification of two different groups,[1] by 1992 the number of complementation groups increased to four.[2] The first FA gene cloned was of complementation group C found to be involved in the correction of DNA cross-links and termed FACC,[3] which was later renamed as FANCC.

Common clinical and cellular phenotypes among different complementation groups led to a hypothesis that the multiple FA gene products function in a single biochemical pathway. This hypothesis was first examined after the second FA gene FANCA was cloned.[4,5] Kupfer et al (1997) reported that FANCA and FANCC form a complex in cytoplasm and translocate into nuclei,[6] although FANCC was previously shown to be predominantly existing in the cytoplasm.[7,8] The nuclear interaction between FANCA and FANCC was disputed by other investigators,[9] but later supported by several independent investigators (see below).

Joenje et al (1997) reported that there are at least 8 complementation groups, FA-A, B, C, D, E, F, G, and H,[10] although FA-H later turned out to be identical with FA-A.[11] These lymphoblast lines of different complementation groups allowed us to examine the above hypothesis for the biochemical pathway(s) constituting multiple FA proteins.[12] In our studies it has been shown that the interaction and nuclear accumulation of FANCA and FANCC are disrupted not only in FA-A and FA-C cells but also in FA-B, E, F, and G, whereas these events are intact in FA-D cells. Based on these findings, a model for the "the FA pathway" has been proposed for FA proteins and their biochemical pathway. According to the model FANCA, B, C, E, F and G interacts in a common pathway and/or complex, whereas FANCD functions downstream or independent of the pathway.[12]

Further evidence for the above model came from cloning of other FA genes. Three FA genes, *FANCG*, *FANCE* and *FANCF* were identified fairly recently as cDNA clones, complementing patient-derived cells.[13-15] Subsequent studies provided evidence that all of these gene products form a complex with FANCA and FANCC (see below) and FANCD2. A gene representing a subgroup of FA-D, was identified very recently[16] Accordingly, a subgroup of FA-D patients without mutations of FANCD2 were assigned into FA-D1. Simultaneous biochemical studies of the FANCD2 protein[17] brought a breakthrough in understanding of the molecular

---

*Takayuki Yamashita—Division of Genetic Diagnosis, Institute of Medical Science, University of Tokyo, Tokyo, Japan. Email: y-taka@showa.gunma-u.ac.jp

Molecular Mechanisms of Fanconi Anemia, edited by Shamim I. Ahmad and Sandra H. Kirk.
©2006 Eurekah.com and Springer Science+Business Media.

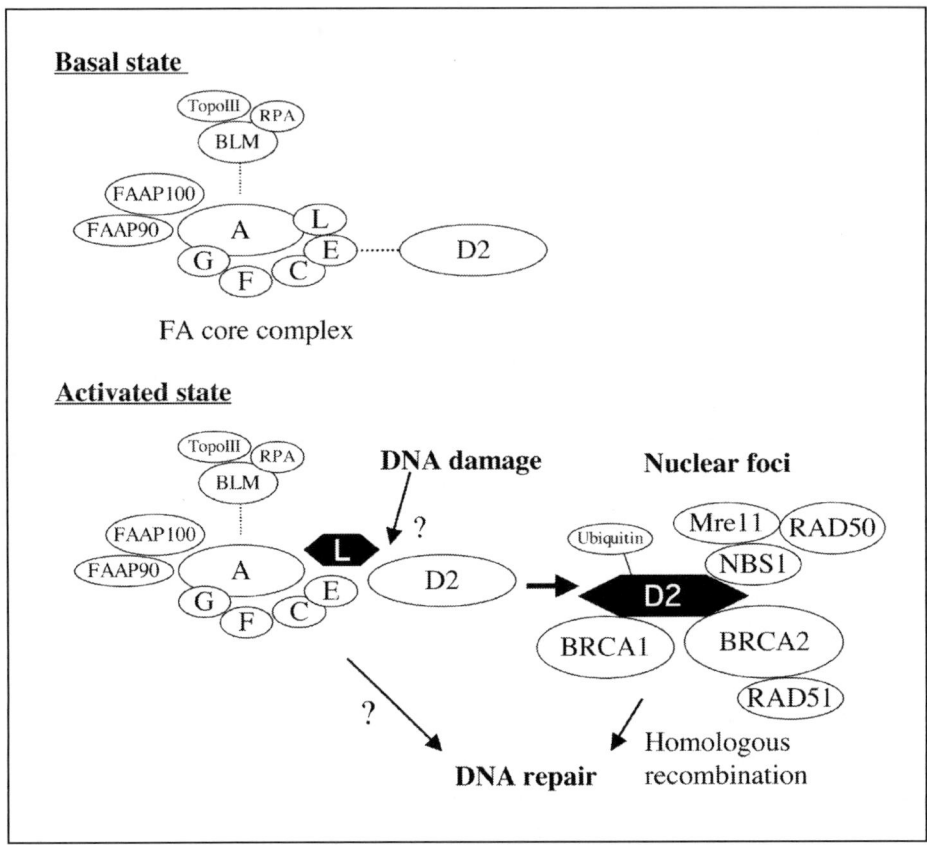

Figure 1. Functions of the FA core complex: a hypothetical model. Topo III:Topoisomerase III, RPA:Replication protein A, A:FANCA, C:FANCC, E:FANCE, F:FANCF, G:FANCG, D2:FANCD2, FAAP:Fanconi anemia-associated polypeptide. See text for details.

mechanisms of the FA pathway: FANCD2 is mono-ubiquitinated to an active form, depending on a multiprotein complex including FANCA, C, E, F and G, now known as the "FA core complex" (Fig. 1). The active isoform of FANCD2 then interacts with BRCA1 in nuclear foci.[17] This finding was further followed by the discovery that FANCD1 is identical with BRCA2.[18] Biallelic mutations of BRCA2 were detected in FA-D1 cells. Moreover, BRCA2 complemented FA-D1 cells. These findings led to the proposed FA/BRCA pathway.[19]

Downstream of the pathway, a mono-ubiquitinated form of FANCD2 interacts with the NBS1/MRE11/RAD50 complex[20] as well as the BRCA1 machinery,[17] both of which play important roles in homologous recombination repair.[21] Null mutations of Brca1 and Brca2 result in embryonic lethality in mice, whereas Fancd2 (-/-) mice show a similar phenotype to Brca2 hypomorphic mice, characterized by chromosome instability, developmental abnormalities and cancer susceptibility.[22] These results suggest that FANCD2 has a modulatory role in the BRCA-mediated homologous recombination. Consistently, FA patients with biallelic mutations of BRCA2 showed much shorter survival than other groups, mainly because of earlier onset of malignancies.[23]

After the finding that mono-ubiquinated FANCD2 interacts with the BRCA1 machinery, attention was focused on an ubiquitin-ligase for FANCD2. None of the previously identified FA proteins, FANCA, C, E, F and G, has been shown to have this enzymatic motif. Since

FANCD2 mono-ubiquitination levels were decreased in BRCA1-deficient cells,[17] BRCA1 was proposed as a possible ubiquitin-ligase involved in the reaction. However, recent studies revealed that BRCA1 is not essential for FANCD2 mono-ubiquitination,[24] although it might enhance the enzymatic activity or stabilize mono-ubiquitinated FANCD2. Biochemical analyses of the immunopurified multiprotein complex, using anti-FANCA antibody, identified a 43-kD core complex-associated protein as a novel ubiquitin-ligase PHF9.[25] Based on complementation analysis it was found that a mutation in the gene PHF9 occurred in a new group of FA patient assigned as group L.[25] This is the first FA gene identified from biochemical analysis of the FA complex as ubiquitin-ligase.

Structure of the FA Core Complex

The interaction of FA proteins was intensively studied by use of coimmunoprecipitation and yeast two-hybrid analyses.[6,12,26-35] These studies indicated that multiple FA proteins interact directly or indirectly to form a multiprotein complex. Recent biochemical analyses of the protein complex, highly immunopurified from the nuclear extracts using anti-FANCA antibody, demonstrated that the nuclear complex contain multiple proteins including at least six FA proteins, FANCA, FANCC, FANCE, FANCF, FANCG and FANCL. In patient-derived cells with biallelic inactivating mutations, mostly with null-mutations of either of FANCA, C, E, F or G, it was found that the interactions between other FA proteins were disrupted.[12,29] Structural basis for the interaction between FANCA and other FA proteins was extensively studied.[33] A number of pathogenic mutations, predicted to produce proteins with amino acid alterations and small in-frame deletions, were found throughout the two-third C-terminal motif of FANCA. These diverse mutations abolished the FANCA interaction with FANCC, FANCF and FANCE in a parallel manner, suggesting that a tertiary rather than local structure of FANCA is important for these interactions.[33]

On the other hand, the FANCA/G interaction was not affected by the absence of other FA proteins or C-terminal mutations of FANCA.[26,27] In vitro binding studies showed that FANCG directly binds to an N-terminal short fragment of FANCA.[26,28] Interestingly, the FANCG-binding region overlaps the bipartite nuclear localizing signal,[26,28,35] which is supposed to bind importin family proteins. Thus, FANCG might regulate nuclear import of FANCA. In an in vitro study the FANCA-binding region of FANCG was mapped to its carboxy-terminus,[28] while in vivo binding study showed that the amino terminal two-thirds section binds to FANCA.[30] Recent studies suggested that some of seven tetratricopeptide repeat motifs of this protein are important for the interaction with FANCA.[36] The yeast 3-hybrid studies suggest that FANCG mediates the interaction between FANCA and FANCF as well as dimerization of FANCA monomers.[34] Consistently, FANCA mutants defective in FANCG binding fail to interact with FANCC, FANCF and FANCE.[26,35] Thus, FANCG may have an integrative role in the FA protein complex.

Direct interactions between FANCC and FANCE and between FANCF and FANCG are detected in yeast 2-hybrid and in vitro binding assays,[31,32] whereas the interaction between FANCF and FANCG is markedly impaired in patient-derived cells lacking other FA proteins.[29] In addition to six known FA proteins, the stable FA core complex contains three unknown FAAPs (Fanconi anemia-associated polypeptide).[25] Identification and characterization of these proteins should provide important information for clarifying the molecular architecture of the core complex.

The FA core complex is intact in FA-D1 and FA-D2 cells,[12,29] indicating that FANCD1/BRCA2 or FANCD2 is not required for the core complex formation. Consistently, these two proteins are not detected in the purified core complex.[25] A mono-ubiquitinated form of FANCD2 interacts with BRCA1 and BRCA2 to form distinct protein complex.[17,37] These observations led to a proposal of a linear model of the FA/BRCA pathway (Fig. 1). On the other hand, recent studies indicate direct interaction between FANCG and BRCA2 and colocalization of FANCG in BRCA2/Rad51 nuclear foci after MMC treatment.[38] Consistently, Rad51 nuclear foci formation is impaired in FA-G cells.[39] Thus, FANCG may directly participate in regulation of the BRCA2/RAD51-mediated homologous recombination, independently of the classical pathway through FANCD2 mono-ubiquitination.

Functions of the FA Core Complex

Most FA proteins in the core complex (FANCA, C, E, F and G) have no enzymatic motif, which is an obstacle to understand their molecular functions. However, FANCL/PHF9, a recently identified 43-kD protein included in the complex, has a PHD-type E3 ubiquitin ligase motif.[25] FANCL/PHF9 has an autoubiquitination activity in vitro. Furthermore, knockdown of this protein using siRNA suppressed FANCD2 mono-ubiquitination and enhanced MMC-induced chromosome breakage. These results indicate that FANCL/PHF9 is a ubiquitin ligase for FANCD2.[25] Since defects of either FA proteins in the core complex abolished FANCD2 mono-ubiquitination,[17,33] protein interactions in the core complex play an important role in the regulation of this enzymatic reaction. However, molecular mechanisms for this regulation are largely unknown but several possibilities can be considered (Fig. 1). First, the core complex appears to be required for nuclear localization of FANCL/PHF9 and nuclear levels of FANCL are reduced in patient-derived cells of multiple complementation groups.[25] Second, the core complex may be required for a proper interaction of FANCL/PHF9 to the substrate FANCD2. In support of this notion, FANCE, a component of the core complex, interacts with FANCD2.[32] Third, active conformation of FANCL/PHF9 might depend on the interactions with other FA proteins in the core complex. Alternatively, the catalytic site of FANCL/PHF9, masked by the core complex might be activated by dissociation from the complex on stimulation.

In a currently proposed model, the preformed core complex is required for the activation of FANCD2. This notion is challenged by our recent observations. An early study demonstrated that, although a Leu25Pro substitution of FANCA N-terminal fragment disrupt the interaction with FANCG in vitro,[28] yet the functional effect of this mutation in vivo was not tested. The mutant protein (Leu25Pro), ectopically expressed in FANCA-null fibroblast, failed to interact with FANCG as well as FANCC, F and E. However, the mutant was predominantly localized in the nuclei, induced FANCD2 mono-ubiquitination and corrected MMC sensitivity.[35] These results suggest that the stable core complex formation is not essential for nuclear localization of FANCA or FANCD2 mono-ubiquitination.

Cell cycle entry into the S phase as well as cellular exposure to various DNA damaging agents including ultraviolet, ionizing radiation, hydroxyurea and DNA crosslinkers induce FANCD2 mono-ubiquitination.[17,40] The induction during the S phase may be attributed to DNA replication-associated strand breaks. How do various kinds of DNA lesions induce FANCD2 mono-ubiquitination? The FA core complex may function as a sensor or a transducer of DNA damage signals leading to the activation of FANCL by changing its subcellular localization and/or conformation. In support for this notion is MMC treatment enhancing association of FANCA, C and G with nuclear matrix and chromosome.[41] Also, it is proposed that alpha-spectrin II recognizes DNA crosslinks, acting as a scaffold to recruit FANCA, C and G proteins to the DNA lesion.[42,43] Alternatively, DNA damage signals may activate FANCD2 by post-translational modification (e.g., phosphorylation) as a target for the catalytic action of FANCL/PHF9.

The FA core complex may directly participate in processing of DNA interstrand crosslinks. Sridharan et al (2003) showed that FANCA associates with XPF,[43] which is thought to be involved in the incision of interstrand crosslinks.[44] This is consistent with previous observations that FA cells are defective in the incision of interstrand crosslinks.[45] In contrast, Rothfuss and Grompe (2004) observed that FA cells are fully proficient in the sensing and incision of interstrand crosslinks and proposed that the FA proteins are involved downstream of the crosslink repair.[46] Meetei et al (2003) showed that BLM, a RecQ helicase responsible for Bloom syndrome, and its associated proteins such as topoisomerase III and replication protein A, weakly interact with the FA core complex,[47] raising the possibility that the FA core complex and the BLM complex collaborate in the processing of DNA damage.

Perspectives

In current model of the FA/BRCA pathway, multiple FA proteins, constituting the core complex, regulate the BRCA machinery-mediated homologous recombination through mono-ubiquitination of FANCD2. This pathway plays an important role in DNA damage response and the maintenance of the genomic integrity. However, the molecular function of the FA core complex FANCA/C/E/F/G/L is poorly understood. An urgent issue is to clarify the regulatory mechanisms for FANCL/PHF9-mediated FANCD2 mono-ubiquitination. A relevant question is what DNA damage signals activate the enzymatic reaction? It is also important to determine whether or not the core complex directly participates in processing of DNA damage. To address these questions, analysis of unknown FA genes, FANCB, I and J,[48] and the core complex-associated proteins (FAAPs)[25,47] is important.

Emerging evidence suggests that acquired inactivation of the FA/BRCA pathway is involved in genomic instability in malignancies. Epigenetic silencing of FANCF was shown in ovarian cancers.[48] Somatic mutations and loss of heterozygosity of FANCC and FANCG were detected in pancreas cancer in young patients.[49] Besides, the somatic inactivation of FA gene expression, abnormal regulation of protein interactions and subcellular distribution of FANCA are suggested to account for defective FANCD2 activation.[50] Various mechanisms can be postulated for the abnormal regulation of the FA/BRCA pathway. Increased expression of negative regulators/inactivators of FA proteins, resulting from viral infection and gene amplification, may perturb the pathway. Another possibility is that stress-induced signals suppress the function of FA proteins through protein modification in a reversible manner. Specifically, the function of FANCA may be regulated by FANCA-binding cytoplasmic serine kinase.[51] Elucidation of the regulatory mechanisms of the FA/BRCA pathway will enhance our understanding of the pathophysiology of genomic instability and cellular response to genotoxic stress.

References

1. Duckworth-Rysiecki G, Cornish K, Clarke CA et al. Identification of two complementation groups in Fanconi anemia. Somat Cell Mol Genet 1985; 11:35-41.
2. Strathdee CA, Duncan AM, Buchwald M. Evidence for at least four Fanconi anaemia genes including FACC on chromosome 9. Nat Genet 1992; 1:196-8.
3. Strathdee CA, Gavish H, Shannon WR et al. Cloning of cDNAs for Fanconi's anaemia by functional complementation. Nature 1992; 356:763-7.
4. Lo Ten Foe JR, Rooimans MA, Bosnoyan-Collins L et al. Expression cloning of a cDNA for the major Fanconi anaemia gene, FAA. Nat Genet 1996; 14:320-3.
5. The Fanconi anaemia/breast cancer consortium. Positional cloning of the Fanconi anaemia group A gene. The Fanconi anaemia/breast cancer consortium. Nat Genet 1996; 14:324-8.
6. Kupfer GM, Naf D, Suliman A et al. The Fanconi anaemia proteins, FAA and FAC interact to form a nuclear complex. Nat Genet 1997; 17:487-490.
7. Yamashita T, Barber DL, Zhu Y et al. The Fanconi anemia polypeptide FACC is localized to the cytoplasm. Proc Natl Acad Sci USA 1994; 91:6712-6.
8. Youssoufian H. Localization of Fanconi anemia C protein to the cytoplasm of mammalian cells. Proc Natl Acad Sci USA 1994; 91:7975-9.
9. Kruyt FA, Youssoufian H. The Fanconi anemia proteins FAA and FAC function in different cellular compartments to protect against cross-linking agent cytotoxicity. Blood 1998; 92:2229-36.
10. Joenje H, Oostra AB, Wijker M et al. Evidence for at least eight Fanconi anemia genes. Am J Hum Genet 1997; 61:940-4.
11. Joenje H, Levitus M, Waisfisz Q et al. Complementation analysis in Fanconi anemia: Assignment of the reference FA-H patient to group A. Am J Hum Genet 2000; 67:759-62.
12. Yamashita T, Kupfer GM, Naf D et al. The Fanconi anemia pathway requires FAA phosphorylation and FAA/FAC nuclear accumulation. Proc Natl Acad Sci USA 1998; 95:13085-13090.
13. de Winter JP, Waisfisz Q, Rooimans MA et al. The Fanconi anaemia group G gene FANCG is identical with XRCC9. Nat Genet 1998; 20:281-283.
14. de Winter JP, Leveille F, van Berkel CG et al. Isolation of a cDNA representing the Fanconi anemia complementation group E gene. Am J Hum Genet 2000; 67:1306-1308.
15. de Winter JP, Rooimans MA, van Der Weel L et al. The Fanconi anaemia gene FANCF encodes a novel protein with homology of ROM. Nat Genet 2000b; 24:15-16.

16. Timmers C, Taniguchi T, Hejna J et al. Positional cloning of a novel Fanconi anemia gene, FANCD2. Mol Cell 2001; 7:241-8.
17. Garcia-Higuera I, Taniguchi T, Ganesan S et al. Interaction of the Fanconi anemia proteins and BRCA1 in a common pathway. Mol Cell 2001; 7:249-62.
18. Howlett NG, Taniguchi T, Olson S et al. Biallelic inactivation of BRCA2 in Fanconi anemia. Science 2002; 297:606-9.
19. D'Andrea AD, Grompe M. The Fanconi anaemia/BRCA pathway. Nat Rev Cancer 2003; 3:23-34.
20. Nakanishi K, Taniguchi T, Ranganathan V et al. Interaction of FANCD2 and NBS1 in the DNA damage response. Nat Cell Biol 2002; 4:913-20.
21. Thompson LH, Schild D. Recombinational DNA repair and human disease. Mutat Res 2002; 509:49-78.
22. Houghtaling S, Timmers C, Noll M et al. Epithelial cancer in Fanconi anemia complementation group D2 (Fancd2) knockout mice. Genes Dev 2003; 17:2021-35.
23. Offit K, Levran O, Mullaney B et al. Shared genetic susceptibility to breast cancer, brain tumors, and Fanconi anemia. J Natl Cancer Inst 2003; 95:1548-51.
24. Vandenberg CJ, Gergely F, Ong CY et al. BRCA1-independent ubiquitination of FANCD2. Mol Cell 2003; 12:247-54.
25. Meetei AR, de Winter JP, Medhurst AL et al. A novel ubiquitin ligase is deficient in Fanconi anemia. Nat Genet 2003; 35:165-70.
26. Garcia-Higuera I, Kuang Y, Naf D et al. Fanconi anemia proteins FANCA, FANCC, and FANCG/XRCC9 interact in a functional nuclear complex. Mol Cell Biol 1999; 19:4866-4873.
27. Waisfisz Q, de Winter JP, Kruyt FA et al. A physical complex of the Fanconi anemia proteins FANCG/XRCC9 and FANCA. Proc Natl Acad Sci USA 1999; 96:10320-10325.
28. Kruyt FA, Abou-Zahr F, Mok H et al. Resistance to mitomycin C requires direct interaction between the Fanconi anemia proteins FANCA and FANCG in the nucleus through an arginine-rich domain. J Biol Chem 1999; 274:34212-8.
29. de Winter JP, van der Weel L, de Groot J et al. The Fanconi anemia protein FANCF forms a nuclear complex with FANCA, FANCC and FANCG. Hum Mol Genet 2000; 9:2665-2674.
30. Kuang Y, Garcia-Higuera I, Moran A et al. Carboxy terminal region of the Fanconi anemia protein, FANCG/XRCC9, is required for functional activity. Blood 2000; 96:1625-32.
31. Medhurst AL, Huber PAJ, Waisfisz Q et al. Direct interactions of the five known Fanconi anaemia proteins suggest a common functional pathway. Hum Mol Genet 2001; 10:423-429.
32. Pace P, Johnson M, Tan WM et al. FANCE: The link between Fanconi anaemia complex assembly and activity. EMBO J 2002; 21:3414-3423.
33. Adachi D, Oda T, Yagasaki H et al. Heterogeneous activation of the Fanconi anemia pathway by patient-derived FANCA mutants. Hum Mol Genet 2002; 11:3125-3134.
34. Gordon SM, Buchwald M. Fanconi anemia protein complex: Mapping protein interactions in the yeast 2- and 3-hybrid systems. Blood 2003; 102:136-41.
35. Adachi T, Oda T, Yagasaki H et al. Stable complex formation of the Fanconi anemia (FA) protein is not essential for activation of the FA pathway. Blood 2003; 100:43a.
36. Blom E, van de Vrugt HJ, de Vries Y et al. Multiple TPR motifs characterize the Fanconi anemia FANCG protein. DNA Repair (Amst) 2004; 3:77-84.
37. Wang X-Z, Andrassen P, D'Andrea AD. Functional interaction of the Fanconi anemia protein, FANCD2, with the breast cancer susceptibility protein, BRCA2, in damaged chromatin. Blood Date 102:159a.
38. Hussain S, Witt E, Huber PA et al. Direct interaction of the Fanconi anaemia protein FANCG with BRCA2/FANCD1. Hum Mol Genet 2003; 12:2503-10.
39. Digweed M, Rothe S, Demuth I et al. Attenuation of the formation of DNA-repair foci containing RAD51 in Fanconi anaemia. Carcinogenesis 2002; 23:1121-6.
40. Taniguchi T, Garcia-Higuera I, Andreassen PR et al. S-phase-specific interaction of the Fanconi anemia protein, FANCD2, with BRCA1 and RAD51. Blood 2002; 100:2414-20.
41. Qiao F, Moss A, Kupfer GM. Fanconi anemia proteins localize to chromatin and the nuclear matrix in a DNA damage- and cell cycle-regulated manner. J Biol Chem 2001; 276:23391-6.
42. McMahon LW, Sangerman J, Goodman SR et al. Human alpha spectrin II and the FANCA, FANCC, and FANCG proteins bind to DNA containing psoralen interstrand cross-links. Biochemistry 2001; 40:7025-34.
43. Sridharan D, Brown M, Lambert WC et al. Nonerythroid alphaII spectrin is required for recruitment of FANCA and XPF to nuclear foci induced by DNA interstrand cross-links. J Cell Sci 2003; 116(Pt 5):823-35.
44. McHugh PJ, Spanswick VJ, Hartley JA. Repair of DNA interstrand crosslinks: Molecular mechanisms and clinical relevance. Lancet Oncol 2001; 2:483-90.

45. Kumaresan KR, Lambert MW. Fanconi anemia, complementation group A, cells are defective in ability to produce incisions at sites of psoralen interstrand cross-links. Carcinogenesis 2000; 21:741-51.
46. Rothfuss A, Grompe M. Repair kinetics of genomic interstrand DNA cross-links: Evidence for DNA double-strand break-dependent activation of the Fanconi anemia/BRCA pathway. Mol Cell Biol 2004; 24:123-34.
47. Meetei AR, Sechi S, Wallisch M et al. A multiprotein nuclear complex connects Fanconi anemia and Bloom syndrome. Mol Cell Biol 2003; 23:3417-26.
48. Levitus M, Rooimans MA, Steltenpool J et al. Heterogeneity in Fanconi anemia: Evidence for two new genetic subtypes. Blood 2003; [10.1182/blood-2003-08-2915].
49. Taniguchi T, Tischkowitz M, Ameziane N et al. Disruption of the Fanconi anemia-BRCA pathway in cisplatin-sensitive ovarian tumors. Nat Med 2003; 9:568-74.
50. van der Heijden MS, Yeo CJ, Hruban RH et al. Fanconi anemia gene mutations in young-onset pancreatic cancer. Cancer Res 2003; 63:2585-8.
51. Lensch MW, Tischkowitz M, Christianson TA et al. Acquired FANCA dysfunction and cytogenetic instability in adult acute myelogenous leukemia. Blood 2003; 102:7-16.
52. Yagasaki H, Adachi D, Oda T et al. A cytoplasmic serine protein kinase binds and may regulate the Fanconi anemia protein FANCA. Blood 2001; 98:3650-7.

CHAPTER 8

Other Proteins and Their Interactions with FA Gene Products

Tetsuya Otsuki and Johnson M. Liu*

Fanconi anemia (FA) is a genetically heterogeneous disorder, consisting of at least nine complementation groups (FA-A, -B, -C, -D1, -D2, -E, -F, -G, -L).[1-3] To date, eight FA genes, FANC-A, -C, -D1 (BRCA2), -D2, -E, -F, -G, -L, have been identified, but the function of each gene product remains unclear. One approach to clarifying these actions is the identification of binding partners, which may yield indirect clues if the biologic function of the binding partner is known. In this chapter, we will review the putative interacting partners of FANCC and FANCA, the first two FA gene products identified.

FANCC-Binding Proteins

Proteins Involved in Oxidative Stress Metabolism: GSTP1 and RED

A number of early reports suggested involvement of reactive oxygen species (ROS) in inducing chromosomal damage and cell death in FA cells.[4,5] Some investigators have also suggested that the sensitivity of FA cells to mitomycin C (MMC) and diepoxybutane (DEB) may be attributed to aberrant redox cycling and oxidative stress.[6] This hypothesis was supported by the observation that glutathione S-transferase P1-1 (GSTP1), which is involved in intracellular detoxification of toxic and carcinogenic substances, binds to FANCC, resulting in an increase in the catalytic activity of GSTP1.[7] Loss of this activation in FA-C cells was found to lead to increased oxidative damage. GSTs are involved in the detoxification of DEB.[8] In addition, it had been reported that wild-type FANCC interacts with and reduces the catalytic activity of NADPH cytochrome P450 reductase (RED), an integral microsomal enzyme that can transfer electrons from NADPH to cytochrome P450 isozymes and cytochrome C.[9] Since MMC is activated by intracellular reduction with RED, FANCC may protect the cell from active MMC by attenuating its activation. Moreover, reduction of RED activity might prevent the generation of ROS, thereby protecting cells from oxidative stress. Taken together, the oxygen-dependent and redox-related sensitivity of FA-C cells to DEB and MMC may be due to the interaction of FANCC with GSTP1 and RED. Recently, FANCG was also reported to bind to cytochrome P450 2E1 (CYP2E1), a member of the P450 superfamily, suggesting a possible role of FANCG in protection against oxidative DNA damage.[10]

Transcriptional Factor and Signal Transducer: FAZF and STAT1

Using the yeast two-hybrid system, Hoatlin et al (1999) identified a novel 486 amino-acid gene product, which was named Fanconi anemia zinc finger (FAZF), as interacting with

*Corresponding Author: Johnson M. Liu, Schneider Children's Hospital, Pediatric Hematology/Oncology and Stem Cell Transplantation, New Hyde Park, New York 11040, U.S.A. Email: jliu3@NSHS.edu

Molecular Mechanisms of Fanconi Anemia, edited by Shamim I. Ahmad and Sandra H. Kirk. ©2006 Eurekah.com and Springer Science+Business Media.

FANCC.[11] FAZF contains three C-terminal zinc finger domains as well as a conserved N-terminal BTB/POZ domain, which is homologous to the promyelocytic leukemia zinc finger protein, PLZF. PLZF was known to act as a transcriptional repressor when associated with nuclear corepressors,[12] and FAZF is thought to act in a similar fashion, binding to the same sequences as PLZF. Since PLZF has an essential role in limb patterning, acting as a growth inhibitory and pro-apoptotic factor in the limb bud,[13] it has been proposed that the FANCC-FAZF interaction may somehow be associated with growth inhibition and developmental anomalies, which are common clinical features of FA.

Other investigators have reported that FA-C cells are hypersensitive to interferon gamma (IFN-γ).[14,15] IFN-γ stimulates activation of the transcription factor STAT1 through docking to activated IFN-γ receptors, resulting in STAT1 phosphorylation.[16] Pang et al (2000) have presented evidence that FANCC binds to STAT1 to aid receptor docking and, in the absence of functional FANCC, STAT1 phosphorylation was not observed. They propose that FANCC plays a role in controlling STAT1-activated transcription, which provides a mitogenic stimulus and activation of apoptotic responses through control of interferon response factor-1. In the absence of FANCC, an imbalance between these pathways might result in apoptosis of hematopoietic progenitor cells and bone marrow failure.[17]

Cell Cycle Regulator: cdc2

Several studies have suggested that FA cells have a molecular defect in cell cycle progression, which has been ascribed to G2 phase arrest.[18,19] For cell cycle progression from G2 to M phase, the cyclin-dependent kinase, cdc2, assembles with cyclin A and cyclin B and phosphorylates multiple substrates in the pathway.[20,21] FANCC was reported to coimmunoprecipitate with cdc2, and expression of FANCC protein appeared to be subject to cell cycle-specific regulation, with peak levels observed at the G2/M transition period.[22]

FANCA-Binding Proteins

From yeast two-hybrid experiments using a C-terminal FANCA fragment as bait, three FANCA-binding proteins, BRG1,[23] IKK2[24] and SNX5,[25] have been identified.

A Component of Chromatin-Remodeling Enzyme Complex: BRG1

BRG1, *brm*-related gene 1, is a key component of the SWI/SNF complex, which remodels chromatin structure through a DNA-dependent ATPase activity.[26] FANCA was demonstrated to associate with the endogenous SWI/SNF complex.[23] Additionally, a significant increase in the molecular chaperone GRP94 was observed among BRG1-associated factors isolated from FANCA-deficient cells, which was not seen in either normal control cells or FANCA-deficient cells complemented by wild-type FANCA. GRP94 was previously identified as a FANCC-binding protein.[27]

As discussed elsewhere, an active form of FANCD2 was found to colocalize with the breast cancer susceptibility protein BRCA1 within ionizing radiation-induced nuclear foci.[28] BRCA1 was initially identified as mutated in patients with familial breast and ovarian cancer, and its putative functions include DNA damage repair,[29] regulation of the G2/M phase checkpoint,[30] and regulation of centrosome duplication.[31] BRCA1 has also been reported to directly interact with BRG1 and is associated with the human SWI/SNF complex.[32] A functional interaction between BRCA1 and BRG1 was suggested by the observation that p53-mediated stimulation of transcription by BRCA1 was completely abrogated by coexpression of a dominant-negative BRG1 mutant.

Interaction between the FA protein complex (FANCA/FANCC/FANCG) and chromatin has been described.[33] According to the report, the FA protein complex was excluded from chromatin of cells in mitosis (M phase), precisely analogous to the behavior of BRG1. Taken together, cell cycle-specific interactions between the chromatin-FA protein complex and between FANCA-BRG1-BRCA1 may allow the repair machinery access to sites of damaged DNA or specific gene targets (Fig. 1).

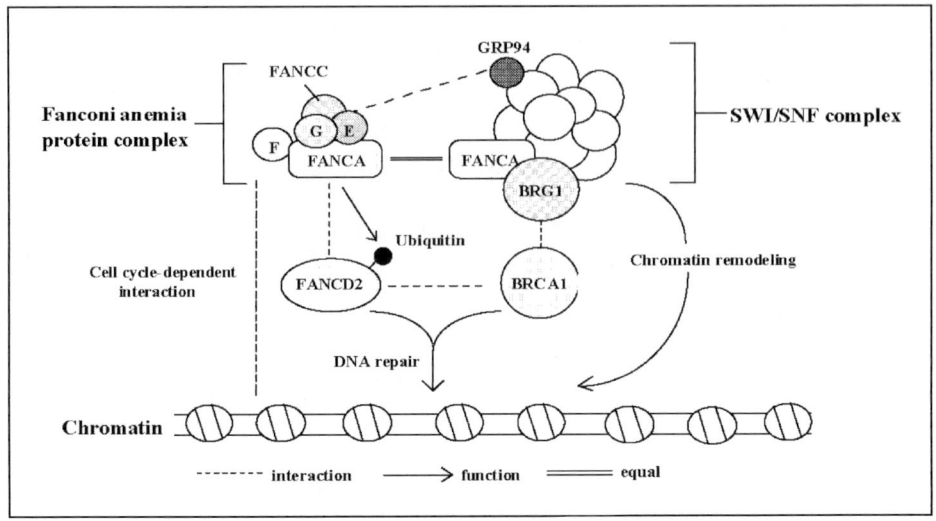

Figure 1. Model of cross-talk between FANCA (FANC protein complex), BRG1 (SWI/SNF complex) BRCA1 and FANCD2.

A Component of IKK Signalsome: IKK2

FA cells have been shown to be hypersensitive to apoptosis induced by tumor necrosis factor-alpha (TNF-α).[34,35] TNF-α mediates this signal through activation of the caspase cascade, whereas an anti-apoptotic signal is concurrently generated by activation of the NF-κB transcription factor.[36,37] NF-κB activation is in turn regulated by proteasomal degradation of inhibitor κB (IκB) by the IκB kinase complex (IKK complex) (Fig. 2). FANCA was recently found to associate with the IKK complex through a direct interaction between FANCA and IKK2, a core component of the IKK complex.[24] In vitro kinase assays suggested that components of the FANCA protein complex are substrates of IKK2. These studies suggest a functional role for the IKK complex in the biological pathway mediated by FANCA. The IKK complex is responsive to both ROS signaling and to DNA damage and exerts its protective effect by activation of NF-κB, resulting in up-regulation of genes involved in redox regulation, DNA repair and resistance to apoptosis.[37] Interaction between FANCA and the IKK complex may therefore explain aberrant apoptosis signaling in FA cells.

Intracellular Trafficking Molecule: SNX5

Among the family of sorting nexins (SNXs), SNX1 was first identified as a protein that bound to the cytoplasmic domain of the epidermal growth factor (EGF) receptor.[38] Based on its homology to a yeast protein (Mvp1p), known to be involved in targeting hydrolases to the vacuole, it was hypothesized that SNX1 was involved in EGF receptor degradation in lysosomes.[39] Over-expression of SNX1 resulted in accelerated degradation of EGF receptor.[38] Subsequently, several proteins were cloned and identified as members of the SNX family on the basis of containing an approximately 100 amino-acid region, termed the phox homology (pX) domain,[40] which is also present in the yeast proteins Mvp1p, Vps5p and Grd19p. All three yeast proteins are involved in intracellular trafficking of target proteins. The pX domain has since been recognized as an interaction domain with phosphoinositide (PI) lipids.[40]

A new member of the SNX family, SNX5 was identified as a binding partner for FANCA,[25] although the functional significance of this association remains unclear. One possibility is that SNX5 is involved in subcellular trafficking of FANCA. FANCA is known to undergo specific

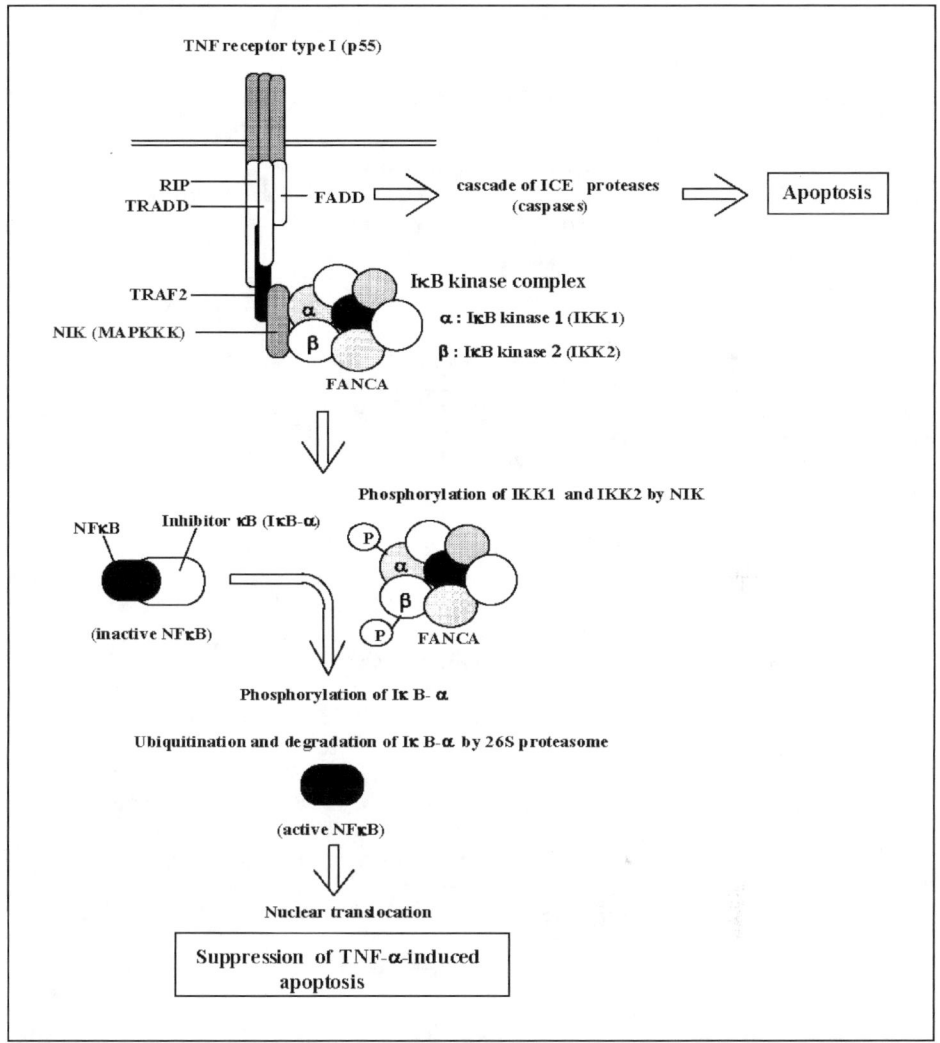

Figure 2. TNF-α signal transduction for activation of NF-κB. FANCA was found to be a component of IKK complex.

phosphorylation, which may be important for its function.[41] Recently, the Akt kinase was reported to regulate FANCA phosphorylation.[42] Remarkably, Akt is a member of a family of protein kinases that contain the pleckstrin homology (pH) domain, which also binds a broad range of PI lipids.[43] These observations suggest that FANCA may be subject to regulation by PI signaling or metabolism.

As an example, phosphoinositide 3-kinase (PI-3K) plays an essential role in Akt activation through the production of phosphatidylinositol-3,4,5-trisphosphate, a lipid second messenger that somehow signals translocation of Akt to the plasma membrane, where it is phosphorylated and activated by phosphoinositide-dependent kinase-1 (PDK-1) and possibly other kinases. It is possible that the interaction between FANCA and SNX5 may localize FANCA to particular subcellular domains, thus subjecting FANCA to regulation by Akt (Fig. 3).

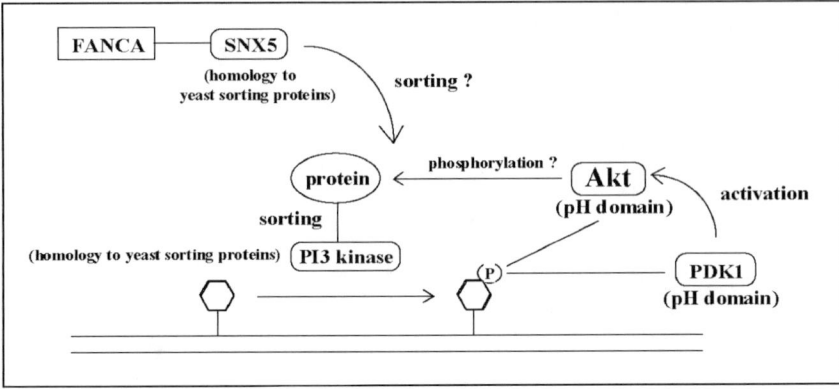

Figure 3. Mechanisms of Akt activation by PDK1 at the site of PtdIns (3) P formation. Both PI3-kinase and SNX5 have homology to yeast sorting proteins, suggesting that FANCA may be sorted by SNX5 for phosphorylation by Akt.

FA Protein Complex and Human α Spectrin II

With regards to assembly of the FA protein complex, human nonerythroid αII spectrin (αSpIIΣ*) has been shown to play an important role.[44] Levels of this protein were reduced in the nuclei of FA cells, and αSpIIΣ* was postulated to act as a scaffold to align or enhance interactions between FA proteins and DNA repair proteins such as ERCC1 and XPF (Fig. 4).

Conclusion

The FA proteins appear to interact with a variety of proteins, and these associations suggest involvement in a number of functions. However, protein components of two major pathways appear more than once in connection with the FA gene products: chromatin remodeling and stress-mediated kinase complexes. There may be cross-talk, for example, between the FA protein complex, the SWI/SNF complex, and the IKK signalsome (Fig. 5). According to this model, the FA protein complex may act to process or repair DNA damage, as a result of interaction with the SWI/SNF complex, BRCA1 and FANCD2, and also modu-

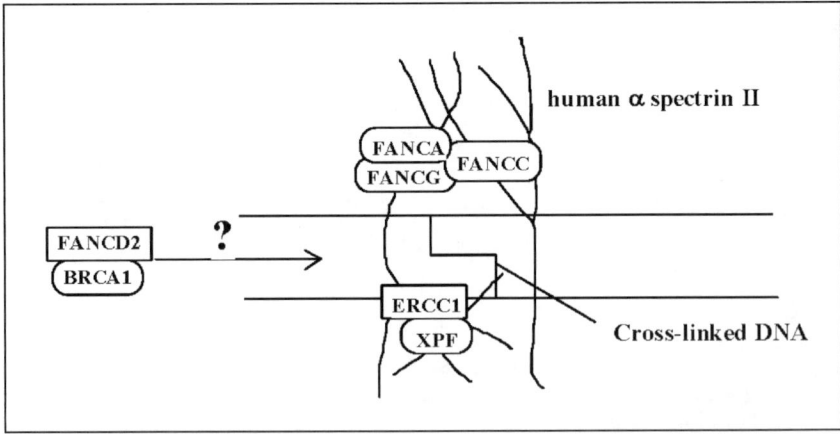

Figure 4. Model of the functional relationship between the FANC protein complex, DNA repair proteins and human α spectrin II.

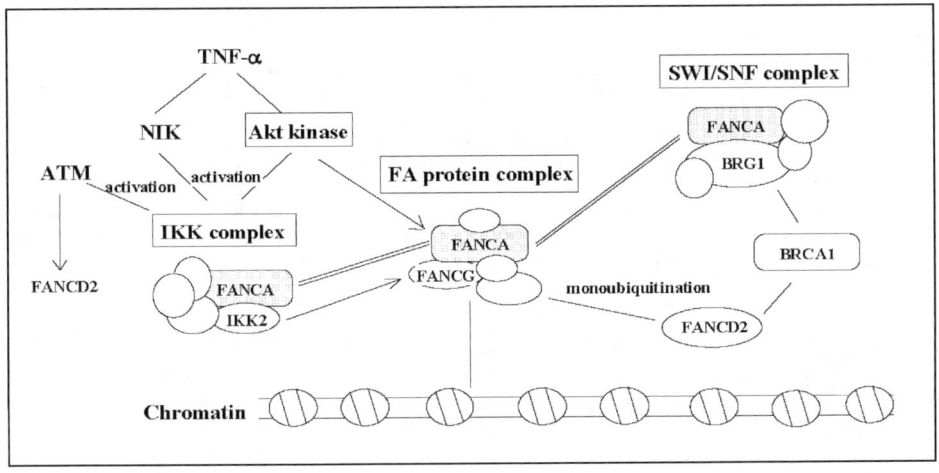

Figure 5. Cross-talk between the FA protein complex, SWI/SNF complex, IKK complex, and Akt. -----: interaction; =====: equal; ----->: phosphorylation.

late apoptosis, through associations with the IKK complex and Akt kinase. The relationship between stress-mediated transcriptional regulation (IKK and NF-κB pathways) and proteins involved in homologous recombination repair (such as BRCA1, BRCA2, etc.) has been well documented[45] and serves to underscore how FA proteins may serve pleiotropic functions. Further investigations will be needed to clarify these various functions and the molecular pathophysiology of FA.

References

1. Joenje H, Levitus M, Waisfisz Q et al. Complementation analysis in Fanconi anemia: Assignment of the reference FA-H patient to group A. Am J Hum Genet 2000; 67:759-762.
2. Timmers C, Taniguchi T, Hejna J et al. Positional cloning of a novel Fanconi anemia gene, FANCD2. Mol Cell 2001; 7:241-248.
3. Joenje H, Patel KJ. The emerging genetic and molecular basis of Fanconi anaemia. Nat Rev Genet 2001; 2:446-457.
4. Nagasawa H, Little JB. Suppression of cytotoxic effect of mitomycin-C by superoxide dismutase in Fanconi's anemia and dyskeratosis congenita fibroblasts. Carcinogenesis 1983; 4:795-799.
5. Ruppitsch W, Meisslitzer C, Hirsch-Kauffmann M et al. Overexpression of thioredoxin in Fanconi anemia fibroblasts prevents the cytotoxic and DNA damaging effect of mitomycin C and diepoxybutane. FEBS Lett 1998; 422:99-102.
6. Pagano G. Mitomycin C and diepoxybutane action mechanisms and FANCC protein functions: Further insights into the role for oxidative stress in Fanconi's anaemia phenotype. Carcinogenesis 2000; 21:1067-1068.
7. Cumming RC, Lightfoot J, Beard K et al. Fanconi anemia group C protein prevents apoptosis in hematopoietic cells through redox regulation of GSTP1. Nat Med 2001; 7:814-820.
8. Vlachodimitropoulos D, Norppa H, Autio K et al. GSTT1-dependent induction of centromerenegative and -positive micronuclei by 1,2:3,4-diepoxybutane in cultured human lymphocytes. Mutagenesis 1997; 12:397-403.
9. Kruyt FA, Hoshino T, Liu JM et al. Abnormal microsomal detoxification implicated in Fanconi anemia group C by interaction of the FAC protein with NADPH cytochrome P450 reductase. Blood 1998; 92:3050-3056.
10. Futaki M, Igarashi T, Watanabe S et al. The FANCG Fanconi anemia protein interacts with CYP2E1: Possible role in protection against oxidative DNA damage. Cacinogenesis 2002; 23:67-72.
11. Hoatlin ME, Zhi Y, Ball H et al. A novel BTB/POZ transcriptional repressor protein interacts with the Fanconi anemia group C protein and PLZF. Blood 1999; 94:3737-3747.
12. Melnick A, Carlile G, Ahmad KF et al. Critical residues within the BTB domain of PLZF and Bcl-6 modulate interaction with corepressors. Mol Cell Biol 2002; 22:1804-1818.

13. Barna M, Hawe N, Niswander L et al. Plzf regulates limb and axial skeletal patterning. Nat Genet 2000; 25:166-172.
14. Whitney MA, Royle G, Low MJ et al. Germ cell defects and hematopoietic hypersensitivity to gamma-interferon in mice with a targeted disruption of the Fanconi anemia C gene. Blood 1996; 88:49-58.
15. Rathbun RK, Faulkner GR, Ostroski MH et al. Inactivation of the Fanconi anemia group C gene augments interferon-gamma-induced apoptotic responses in hematopoietic cells. Blood 1997; 90:974-985.
16. Pang Q, Fagerlie S, Christianson TA et al. The Fanconi anemia protein FANCC binds to and facilitates the activation of STAT1 by gamma interferon and hematopoietic growth factors. Mol Cell Biol 2000; 20:4724-4735.
17. Pang Q, Keeble W, Christianson TA et al. FANCC interacts with Hsp70 to protect hematopoietic cells from IFN-gamma/TNF-alpha-mediated cytotoxicity. EMBO J 2001; 20:4478-4489.
18. Dutrillaux B, Aurias A, Dutrillaux AM et al. The cell cycle of lymphocytes in Fanconi anemia. Hum Genet 1982; 62:327-332.
19. Kaiser TN, Lojewski A, Dougherty C et al. Flow cytometric characterization of the response of Fanconi's anemia cells to mitomycin C treatment. Cytometry 1982; 2:291-297.
20. Moreno S, Hayles J, Nurse P. Regulation of p34cdc2 protein kinase during mitosis. Cell 1989; 58:361-372.
21. Ducommun B, Brambilla P, Felix MA et al. cdc2 phosphorylation is required for its interaction with cyclin. EMBO J 1991; 10:3311-3319.
22. Kupfer GM, Yamashita T, Naf D et al. The Fanconi anemia polypeptide, FAC, binds to the cyclin-dependent kinase, cdc2. Blood 1997; 90:1047-1054.
23. Otsuki T, Furukawa Y, Ikeda K et al. Fanconi anemia protein, FANCA, associates with BRG1, a component of the human SWI/SNF complex. Hum Mol Genet 2001; 10:2651-2660.
24. Otsuki T, Young DB, Sasaki DT et al. Fanconi anemia protein complex is a novel target of the IKK signalsome. J Cell Biochem 2002; 86:613-623.
25. Otsuki T, Kajigaya S, Ozawa K et al. SNX5, a new member of the sorting nexin family, binds to the Fanconi anemia complementation group A protein. Biochem Biophys Res Commun 1999; 265:630-635.
26. Khavari PA, Peterson CL, Tamkun JW et al. BRG1 contains a conserved domain of the SWI2/SNF2 family necessary for normal mitotic growth and transcription. Nature 1993; 366:170-174.
27. Hoshino T, Wang J, Devetten MP et al. Molecular chaperone GRP94 binds to the Fanconi anemia group C protein and regulates its intracellular expression. Blood 1998; 91:4379-4386.
28. Garcia-Higuera I, Taniguchi T, Ganesan S et al. Interaction of the Fanconi anemia proteins and BRCA1 in a common pathway. Mol Cell 2001; 7:249-262.
29. Chen Y, Lee WH, Chew HK. Emerging roles of BRCA1 in transcriptional regulation and DNA repair. J Cell Physiol 1999; 181:385-392.
30. Deng CX, Scott F. Role of the tumor suppressor gene Brca1 in genetic stability and mammary gland tumor formation. Oncogene 2000; 19:1059-1064.
31. Xu X, Weaver Z, Linke SP et al. Centrosome amplification and a defective G2-M cell cycle checkpoint induce genetic instability in BRCA1 exon 11 isoform-deficient cells. Mol Cell 1999; 3:389-395.
32. Bochar DA, Wang L, Beniya H et al. BRCA1 is associated with a human SWI/SNF-related complex: Linking chromatin remodeling to breast cancer. Cell 2000; 102:257-265.
33. Qiao F, Moss A, Kupfer GM. Fanconi anemia proteins localize to chromatin and the nuclear matrix in a DNA damage- and cell cycle-regulated manner. J Biol Chem 2001; 276:23391-23396.
34. Haneline LS, Broxmeyer HE, Cooper S et al. Multiple inhibitory cytokines induce deregulated progenitor growth and apoptosis in hematopoietic cells from Fac-/- mice. Blood 1998; 91:4092-4098.
35. Otsuki T, Nagakura S, Wang J et al. Tumor necrosis factor-alpha and CD95 ligation suppress erythropoiesis in Fanconi anemia C gene knockout mice. J Cell Physiol 1999; 179:79-86.
36. Mercurio F, Zhu H, Murray BW et al. IKK-1 and IKK-2: Cytokine-activated IkappaB kinases essential for NF-kappaB activation. Science 1997; 278:860-866.
37. Mercurio F, Manning AM. NF-kappaB as a primary regulator of the stress response. Oncogene 1999; 18:6163-6171.
38. Kurten RC, Cadena DL, Gill GN. Enhanced degradation of EGF receptors by a sorting nexin, SNX1. Science 1996; 272:1008-1010.
39. Horazdovsky BF, Davies BA, Seaman MN et al. A sorting nexin-1 homologue, Vps5p, forms a complex with Vps17p and is required for recycling the vacuolar protein-sorting receptor. Mol Biol Cell 1997; 8:1529-1541.
40. Xu Y, Seet LF, Hanson B et al. The Phox homology (PX) domain, a new player in phosphoinositide signalling. Biochem J 2001; 360:513-530.

41. Yamashita T, Kupfer GM, Naf D et al. The fanconi anemia pathway requires FAA phosphorylation and FAA/FAC nuclear accumulation. Proc Natl Acad Sci USA 1998; 95:13085-13090.
42. Otsuki T, Nagashima T, Komatsu N et al. Phosphorylation of fanconi anemia protein, FANCA, is regulated by Akt kinase. Biochem Biophys Res Commun 2002; 291:628-634.
43. Itoh T, Takenawa T. Phosphoinositide-binding domains: Functional units for temporal and spatial regulation of intracellular signalling. Cell Signal 2002; 14:733-743.
44. McMahon LW, Sangerman J, Goodman SR et al. Human alpha spectrin II and the FANCA, FANCC, and FANCG proteins bind to DNA containing psoralen interstrand cross-links. Biochemistry 2001; 40:7025-7034.
45. Thompson LH, Schild D. Recombinational DNA repair and human disease. Mutat Res 2002; 509:49-78.

CHAPTER 9

Fanconi Anaemia and Oxidative Stress:
Cellular and Clinical Phenotypes

Giovanni Pagano* and Shamim I. Ahmad

Abstract

The cellular and clinical phenotypes of Fanconi Anaemia (FA) have been associated with a set of redox abnormalities using evidence arising from in vitro, in vivo and molecular studies. The available information points to: (i) the influence of oxygen and antioxidants in chromosomal instability and in apoptosis; (ii) the redox-related toxicity mechanisms of agents (commonly termed "crosslinkers") triggering excess sensitivity of FA cells; (iii) a set of abnormalities in redox biomarkers detected in body fluids and blood cells from FA patients; (iv) a number of clinical features related to a chronic pro-oxidant state, and (v) the involvement of redox pathways in the functions and structures of at least three proteins encoded by FA genes (FANCA, FANCC and FANCG). Oxidative stress may thus be envisaged as an important phenomenon in FA accounting for most of the findings observed in FA's clinical phenotype. This information ought to prompt clinical studies that might unveil new avenues in FA research, such as the prospect of controlled chemoprevention trials aimed at counteracting the FA-associated pro-oxidant state and ameliorating FA's clinical course.

Introduction

The Oxidative Stress Theory: Historical Background

Most scientific research on FA points to a deficiency in DNA repair in response to DNA damage. The damage can be endogenous or induced by exogenous agents such as mitomycin C (MMC), diepoxybutane (DEB), cis-platin, cyclophosphamide, hexavalent chromium compounds and 8-methoxypsoralen plus near ultraviolet light (PUVA).[1-9] However, the sensitivities of FA cells to MMC and DEB have also been attributed to interference with the redox cycle and point to a role of oxidative stress in the onset of the disease.[10-12] This chapter aims to support the "Oxidative Stress Theory" in FA and its relevance in explaining the composite FA clinical phenotype. Apart from bone marrow failure and susceptibility to haematological and nonhaematological malignancies, FA is also characterized by a set of malformations and abnormalities including type II diabetes mellitus, other endocrine abnormalities and altered skin pigmentation.[13] An endogenous pro-oxidant state[14] is proposed here as the central event accounting for the multiple clinical patterns observed in FA.

Nordenson was the first to report a link between a redox imbalance and FA phenotype by showing a decrease in chromosomal instability of FA cells exposed to antioxidant enzymes.[15] Thereafter, a number of studies have pointed to a pro-oxidant state in FA, including data from in vitro, in vivo and molecular studies.[16] Ostrakhovitch and Afanas'ev[17] showed that the natural

*Corresponding Author: Giovanni Pagano—Centre for Research, Innovation and Technology Transfer in Oncology and Life Sciences, I-83013 Mercogliano (AV), Italy. Email: gbpagano@tin.it

Molecular Mechanisms of Fanconi Anemia, edited by Shamim I. Ahmad and Sandra H. Kirk. ©2006 Eurekah.com and Springer Science+Business Media.

bioflavonoid rutin (vitamin P) inhibited reactive oxygen species (ROS) overproduction in FA, previously reported by Korkina et al.[10] Publications referring to oxidative stress in FA remain a minority in the FA literature, but since 1998 reports have appeared that at least three FA proteins have direct implications in redox pathways.[12,18-20]

Diagnosis and Toxicity Mechanisms of FA-Related Xenobiotics

FA diagnosis is performed by assessing excessive cellular sensitivity to two clastogens, DEB and MMC which interact with DNA and bring about chromosomal instability.[3] The sensitivity of FA cells to these agents is commonly referred to as "crosslinker-sensitivity".[3,7] This term relates to the formation of DNA crosslinks as an ultimate outcome of DEB and MMC toxicity.[21-24] The experimental findings that FA cells are unable to repair DNA crosslinks has led to the current opinion that FA phenotype results from defective responses to DNA damage.[2,7] Here it is argued that the toxicity of these xenobiotics involve redox-dependent mechanisms, suggesting an endogenous deficiency in FA cells in coping with exogenous sources of oxidative stress.[12,14,21-39]

Propensity of Cells to DNA Crosslinking Agents and Oxidative Stress

Mitomycin C

A well studied end product of mitomycin C (MMC) is a DNA adduct.[3,21-23,34] However, the activation of MMC also involves generation of ROS, specifically hydroxyl radicals ($\cdot$OH) and semiquinone radicals via a series of redox reactions.[21-23,34,36,37] The MMC interaction with DNA, furthermore, is dependent on O_2 levels[38,39] and is counteracted by certain ROS scavenging enzymes, superoxide dismutase (SOD) and catalase[30] and by over-expression of thioredoxin pointing to a role for abnormal redox activity.[40]

Diepoxybutane

Similar to MMC, the sensitivity of FA cell lines to diepoxybutane (DEB) can also be attributed to redox associated mechanisms due to the following reasons: (i) its toxicity correlates to oxygen levels;[39] (ii) the epoxide structure of DEB points to a scavenging role vis a vis glutathione (GSH),[24] and (iii) DEB exposure of cells results in depletion of GSH;[39] (iv) GSH depletion in GSST-1 null mutant cells (mutated in glutathione S-transferase T1 gene) results in increased toxicity to DEB[41] and micronucleus formation[42] and, finally, (v) the reduction of DEB induced toxicity in human lymphocytes expressing GSST1 and by thioredoxin (Trx) over-expression.[40,41]

Cyclophosphamide

A report by Joenje and Oostra showed that FA cells are sensitive to cyclophosphamide (CP), which enhances chromosomal instability without S-9 metabolic activation, suggesting a constitutive expression of phase 1 activities for xenobiotic biotransformation.[28] In nonFA cells, CP is known to be an inactive agent, which must first undergo biotransformation to an active metabolite.[43,44] The toxicity of CP is associated with lipid peroxidation and this can be counteracted by alpha-tocopherol.[44] These results, also, point to an involvement of a prooxidant state in FA cells.

Cisplatin

Platinum compounds such as cis-platin (CDDP) are also highly cytotoxic to FA cells[6] which is attributed to their crosslinking with DNA. However, CDDP has first to be activated via a cascade of redox associated biotransformation events.[45,46] Also nephrotoxicity has been shown to be associated with the induction of heme oxygenase[46] and the cellular toxicity induced by CDDP has been shown to be counteracted by antioxidants, such as vitamin C, alpha-tocopherol and N-acetylcysteine.[45,47]

An involvement of redox abnormalities in FA was suggested by a report showing over-expression of p21$^{wafl/cip1}$ in FA lymphoblasts, and its expression was further enhanced by CDDP.[48] Proposed roles of p21$^{wafl/cip1}$ are: oxidative stress regulation,[49] G1 cell cycle arrest and G2 cell cycle regulation.

8-Methoxypsoralen Plus Ultraviolet A

PUVA was one of the earliest agents FA cells were shown to be sensitive to.[5,50] This sensitivity has been associated with crosslinking of the psoralen molecule with DNA in the presence of UVA. However, other mechanisms of PUVA action may also be in operation since direct and indirect evidence is available that shows PUVA may also act upon DNA via ROS. By EPR (electron paramagnetic resonance) analysis, it has been shown that UVA photolysis of this compound can produce ROS.[51] Also PUVA can induce formation of 8-OHdG (8-hydroxy deoxy guanosine) in DNA, indicative of ROS mediated reactions.[52] PUVA also causes GSH depletion leading to oxidative stress conditions.[53] Other researchers favoured another mode of action of PUVA on cells by showing that this agent can damage membranes and proposed that an additional reason for FA cell sensitivity may be lipid peroxidation via ROS formation.[54]

Hexavalent Chromium

FA cells are also sensitive to Cr(VI).[8] Evidence has been presented that indicates Cr(VI) toxicity of FA cells involves multiple redox related events including depletion of glutathione and other thiol based antioxidants.[55,56] Other studies confirmed this by showing protective effects of catalase, melatonin and N-acetylcysteine[57,58] on lipid peroxidation and Cr(VI)-induced ROS formation.[58-60] It is likely that the final stage of Cr(VI) binding to DNA occurs via a cascade of reactions, one of which includes redox dependent mechanisms.

FA Proteins Involvement in Redox Pathways

The protein encoded by FANCC has been shown to associate with other proteins having recognized redox activities, namely NADPH cytochrome P450 reductase[20] and glutathione S-transferase.[18] Moreover, FANCG protein interacts with cytochrome P450 2E1,[19] an activity known to be involved in redox biotransformation of xenobiotics. FANCA and FANCG proteins have also recently been demonstrated to respond to redox state in terms of physical structure and associated with their ability to form disulfide bonds in the FA protein complex.[61] Thus, at least FANCA and FANCG seem to be directly influenced by redox status. Using a yeast two-hybrid study, Reuter et al reported on 69 proteins interacting with FANCA, FANCC, or FANCG proteins.[31] Some of these proteins are involved in transcriptional regulation, cell signalling, oxidative metabolism, and intracellular transport.[31,33] By using oligonucleotide microarrays, Zanier et al showed consistent differential patterns of expression between FANCC mutated and corrected cells.[33] A total of 49 RNAs were isolated which showed a dramatic over-expression of a set of proteins including Nuclear Factor 1 (expressed 26-fold higher in fancc -/- cells), 70kDa heat shock protein (4.5-fold) and cyclooxygenase 2 (3.6-fold). Therefore, at least for these proteins, a consistent body of evidence relates to the induction of a pro-oxidant state in FA. Also it is worth noting that no changes were detected in the expression of any of the DNA repair related activities investigated in these studies.[33]

Altogether, studies on FANCA, FANCC and FANCG proteins provide evidence for their roles in redox-related activities, and to a unique functional and structural sensitivity to redox status.[18-20,31,33,61] The implications of FANCC or FANCG deficiency in redox pathways and phenotypic abnormalities are shown in Figure 1, that include, among others, glutathione imbalance and oxidation of biomolecules (DNA, amino acids and carbohydrates), consistent with some major clinical features, unconfined to bone marrow failure and malignancies, including the endocrinopathies.[13,62]

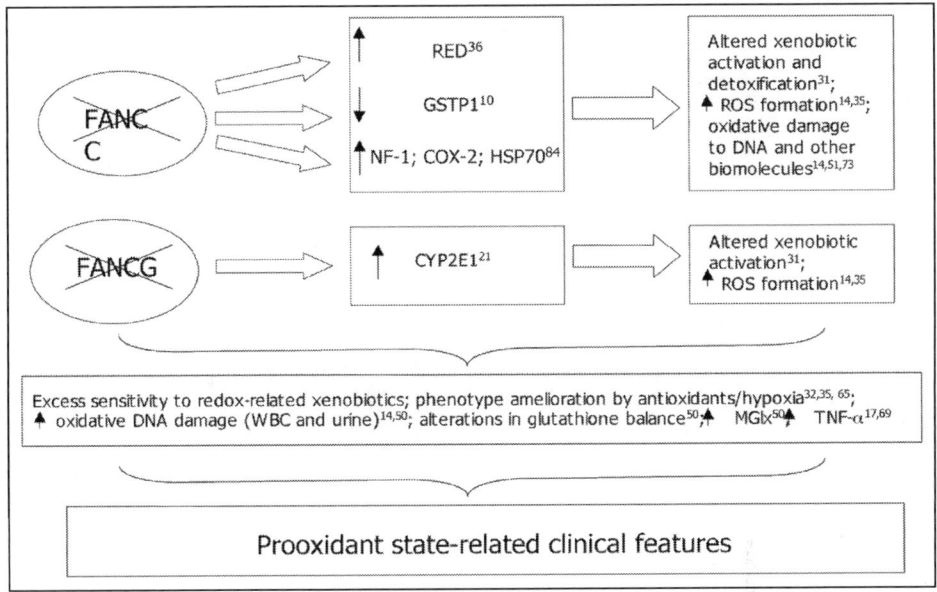

Figure 1. Defective FANCC or FANCG expression lead to a set of imbalances in redox pathways that, in turn, are suggested to cause a prooxidant state at the cellular and at the organismal level.

In Vitro and in Vivo Evidence for a Pro-Oxidant State in FA

FA is characterized by: (i) excessive levels of 8-OHdG on H_2O_2-exposure indicating susceptibility to oxidative DNA damage;[32] (ii) increased 8-OHdG levels in peripheral white blood cells, correlating with spontaneous chromosomal instability, and also expressing excess luminol-dependent chemiluminescence;[10,25,26] (iii) a significant increase in 8-OHdG in the urine, denoting an in vivo proficiency for removing and excreting damaged DNA bases;[26] (iv) increased sensitivity to oxygen and free iron;[28,35] (v) excess plasma levels of clastogenic factor, tumor necrosis factor-α (TNF-α)[66,67] and interferon-γ (IFN-γ);[27,68] (vi) an involvement of thioredoxin, which corrects MMC and DEB sensitivity in FA cells, and is present in lower-than-normal levels in FA fibroblasts.[40,69] An important feature is the correction of chromosomal abnormalities[15,63,64] and of apoptotic propensity[65] by either antioxidant enzymes or by low molecular weight antioxidants.

Together, a well-established body of evidence on the FA phenotype reveals a major role for oxidative stress, while the data on increased 8-OHdG urinary excretion[26] stand against a deficiency in removing oxidatively damaged DNA bases. Takeuchi and Morimoto showed that decomposition of H_2O_2 in FA-A cells was 20-30% decreased and suggested that at least FA-A cells are more prone to oxidative DNA damage most likely due to lowering of catalase activity.[32] In a recent study Pearl-Yafe's group showed that FA-C cells are highly sensitive to IFN-γ and are more sensitive to oxidative stress than FA-A cells.[68]

A Composite Clinical Phenotype: Seeking a Unified Frame

The redox-related information on the FA phenotypes raises the as yet open question about the involvement of oxidative stress in the clinical features and progression of the disease. A number of other abnormalities and complications are observed in FA patients, including: (a) myelogenous leukaemias and a set of solid tumours;[1] (b) malformations of various organs;[2] (c) anomalies in skin pigmentation,[2] and (d) a set of endocrine abnormalities.[13] The most common endocrinopathies, occurring in over 80% of FA patients, include: (i) hyperglycaemia,

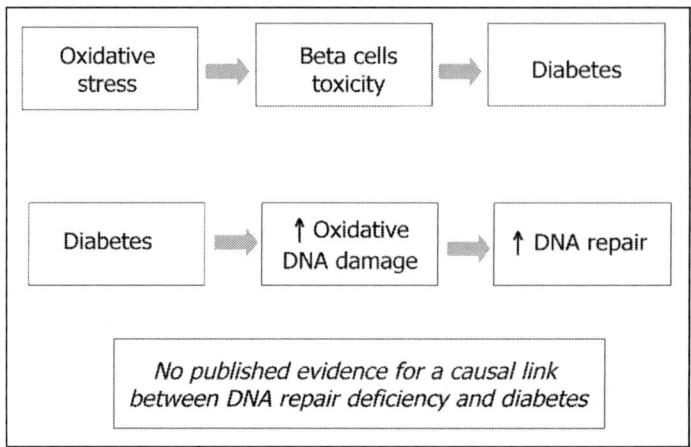

Figure 2. Relationships of: 1) oxidative stress as a diabetogenic agent; 2) diabetes as causing oxidative DNA damage and then upregulation of DNA repair systems. No relationship can be found in the literature for any deficiency in DNA repair as a direct or indirect cause of diabetes. Modified from Pagano et al, 2005.[11]

glucose intolerance and hyperinsulinaemia up to overt diabetes mellitus, (ii) growth hormone (GH) insufficiency, and (iii) hypothyroidism.[13] The literature provides extensive evidence for links between oxidative stress and diabetes pathogenesis, as shown in Figure 2. To the best of our knowledge, no plausible explanation has been provided for these clinical features observed in FA (see Fig. 2). Here we propose a link between the FA clinical phenotype, including the progression to pancytopenia and malignancies as well as some of the "side" clinical complications and features to oxidative stress as an aetiological factor in FA pathogenesis.

Bone marrow failure is known to be caused by several physical (e.g., radiation[70]) and chemical agents (such as benzene[71]) responsible for generating ROS. Thus due to the recognized sensitivity of bone marrow to oxidative stress, it may be suggested that an endogenous pro-oxidant state may result in the haematopoietic failure observed in FA.

Somewhat less pronounced, yet consistent results relate oxidative stress to other clinical features seen in FA patients. The abnormalities in skin pigmentation (*café-au-lait* spots) seen in FA patients can be explained by redox-related molecular mechanisms, as melanin biosynthesis involves an oxidation process.[72,73] A link between melanogenesis and FA was provided by a report relating Trx expression to melanin biosynthesis.[40,74,75] The Trx system in FA cells may thus be regarded both as a component accounting for a pro-oxidant state, and as a mechanistic link for abnormalities in skin pigmentation.

Malformations of various organs occurring in FA patients can also be associated with prenatal exposure to a redox imbalance.[76] Several mechanisms of action of teratogens include ROS formation via their bioactivation by cytochrome P450, prostaglandin H synthase and lipoxygenases to electrophilic and/or free radical reactive intermediates that covalently bind to or oxidize cellular macromolecules such as DNA, proteins and lipids.[76] A noteworthy analogy may be found between the prevailing deformations of forelimbs in FA and in thalidomide-associated teratogenesis. Thalidomide has been reported to induce oxidative stress and glutathione depletion in the nuclei of limb bud cells from rabbit (a sensitive species) more markedly compared to rat (an insensitive species).[77]

An evaluation of the literature available in MedLine (mid-December 2004) was made by combining the key-words related to the major features seen in FA vs. the terms "oxidative stress" and "DNA repair". As shown in Figure 3, the term "DNA repair" is found in the vast majority of publications regarding "chromosomal instability" (221 citations), compared to "oxidative stress" (27 citations). Likewise, for "bone marrow failure", "leukaemia and cancer", and

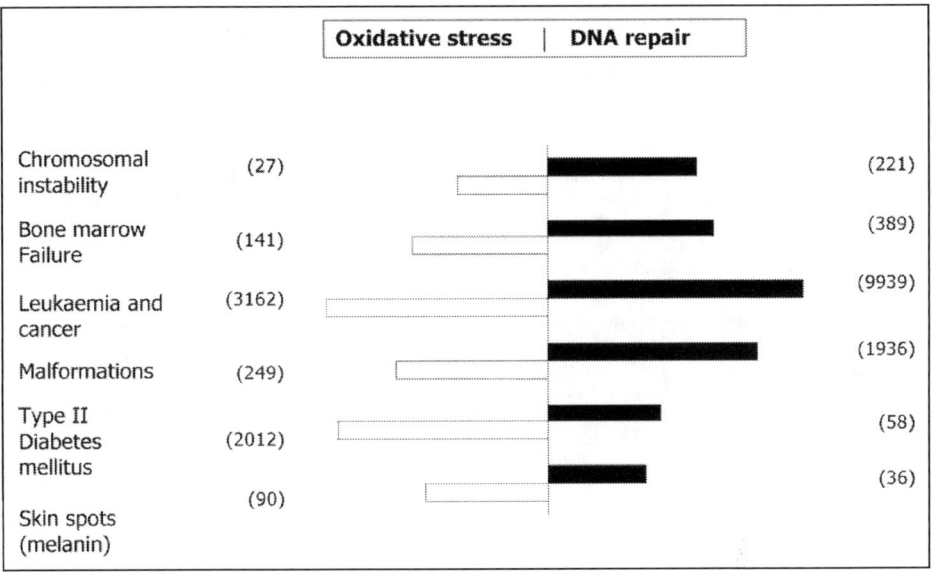

Figure 3. Numbers of journal papers (MedLine, December 2004) associating the major cellular or clinical features seen in FA vs. the key-terms "DNA repair" and "oxidative stress".

"malformations", most of the citations match the term "DNA repair", though lesser, yet substantial numbers of citations are associated with "oxidative stress". On the contrary, the terms "diabetes" and "melanin" ("skin spots") are mostly associated with "oxidative stress". Some reports provided evidence for upregulation of DNA repair systems both in diabetes[78,79] and in melanin biosynthesis.[80,81] None of the citations found for these terms referred to any causative role of DNA repair in diabetes or in melanin formation. In summary, the literature provides a substantial body of evidence supporting a crucial role for oxidative stress in all of the biological and clinical features of FA. On the other hand, a DNA repair deficiency theory may be associated with chromosomal instability, cancer proneness and bone marrow failure, yet there is a lack of plausible evidence accounting for its involvement in certain "side" features seen in FA, including diabetes and skin spots.

Conclusion

In an attempt to evaluate the fitness of a theory in accounting for the observed phenomena, the scientific community is faced with the dilemma of whether the multiple outcomes in the FA phenotype better reflect the scenarios of a deficiency in response to DNA damage,[2,3,7,9] or an impaired redox state leading to a number of cellular and clinical features, as is discussed here. We may envisage the FA-associated clinical pattern as a set of endogenous events resulting in a combined series of pathologies, and/or of abnormalities in redox endpoints. An additional role has been reported for BRCA2 in repairing oxidatively damaged DNA,[82] while FANCD2 monoubiquitination has been reported to depend on ATR checkpoint kinase.[83] These two proteins have been shown to play major roles in DNA repair pathways,[7,9,84] yet they have direct implications in redox pathways including p53, which is upregulated by oxidative stress,[85] and p21,$^{waf1/cip1}$ being active as an oxidative stress sensor.[49] No other explanation is available which gives a sound mechanistic link between response to DNA damage (or DNA repair) and the multiple phenotypic features seen in various FA cell lines and in FA patients.

In conclusion, the current state-of-the-art may prompt the medical community to recognize that the evidence accumulated so far should lead to an appraisal of FA as an oxidative stress-related disorder. This new definition might help to sort out the present maze of «multiple symptoms and complications» in a unifying interpretation of FA, with possible implications on the design of clinical studies leading to real advancement in patients' management.

References

1. Alter BP. Fanconi anemia and malignancies. Am J Hematol 1996; 53:99-110.
2. Alter BP. Fanconi anaemia and its variability. Brit J Haematol 1993; 85:9-14.
3. Auerbach AD, Wolman SR. Susceptibility of Fanconi anaemia fibroblasts to chromosome damage by carcinogens. Nature 1976; 261:494-496.
4. Ishida R, Buchwald M. Susceptibility of Fanconi anemia lymphoblasts to DNA cross-linking and alkylating agents. Cancer Res 1982; 42:4000-4006.
5. Moustacchi E, Diatloff-Zito C. DNA semiconservative synthesis in normal and Fanconi anemia fibroblasts following treatment with 8-methoxypsoralen and near ultraviolet light or with x-rays. Hum Genet 1985; 70:236-242.
6. Poll EH, Arwert F, Joenje H et al. Cytogenetic toxicity of anti-tumor platinum compounds in Fanconi's anemia. Hum Genet 1982; 61:228-230.
7. Taniguchi T, D'Andrea AD. Molecular pathogenesis of Fanconi anemia. Int J Hematol 2002; 75:123-128.
8. Vilcheck SK, O'Brien TJ, Pritchard DE et al. Fanconi anemia complementation group A cells are hyper-sensitive to chromium (IV) induced toxicity. Environ Health Perspect 2002; 110(Suppl 5):773-777.
9. Wang X, D'Andrea AD. The interplay of Fanconi anemia proteins in the DNA damage response. DNA Repair (Amst) 2004; 3:1063-1069.
10. Korkina LG, Samochatova EV, Maschan AA et al. Release of active oxygen radicals by leukocytes of Fanconi's anemia patients. J Leukocyte Biol 1992; 52:357-62.
11. Pagano G, Degan P, d'Ischia M et al. Oxidative stress as a multiple effector in Fanconi anaemia clinical phenotype. Eur J Haematol 2005; 75:93-100.
12. Pagano G, Youssoufian H. Fanconi's anaemia proteins: Concurrent roles in cell protection against oxidative damage. BioEssays 2003; 25:589-595.
13. Wajnrajch MP, Gertner JM, Huma Z et al. Evaluation of growth and hormonal status in patients referred to the International Fanconi Anemia Registry. Paediatrics 2001; 107:744-754.
14. Gille JJ, Wortelboer HM, Joenje H. Antioxidant status of Fanconi anemia fibroblasts. Hum Genet 1987; 77:28-31.
15. Nordenson I. Effect of superoxide dismutase and catalase on spontaneously occuring chromosome breaks in patients with Fanconi's anemia. Hereditas 1977; 86:147-150.
16. Bogliolo M, Cabre O, Callen E et al. The Fanconi anemia genome stability and tumour suppressor network. Mutagenesis 2002; 17:529-538.
17. Ostrakhovitch EA, Afanas'ev IB. Oxidative stress in rheumatoid arthritis leukocytes: Suppression by rutin and other antioxidants and chelators. Biochem Pharmacol 2001; 62:743-746.
18. Cumming RC, Lightfoot J, Beard K et al. Fanconi anemia group C protein prevents apoptosis in hematopoietic cells through redox regulation of GSTP1. Nature Med 2001; 7:814-20.
19. Futaki M, Igarashi T, Watanabe S et al. The FANCG Fanconi anemia protein interacts with CYP2E1: Possible role in protection against oxidative DNA damage. Carcinogenesis 2002; 23:67-72.
20. Kruyt FA, Hoshino T, Liu JM et al. Abnormal microsomal detoxification implicated in Fanconi anemia group C by interaction of the FAC protein with NADPH cytochrome P450 reductase. Blood 1998; 92:3050-3056.
21. Dusre L, Rajagopalan S, Eliot HM et al. DNA interstrand cross-link and free radical formation in a human multidrug resistant cell line from mitomycin C and its analogues. Cancer Res 1990; 50:648-652.
22. Gutteridge JMC, Quinlan GJ, Wilkins S. Mitomycin C-induced deoxyribose degradation inhibited by superoxide dismutase. A reaction involving iron, hydroxyl and semiquinone radicals. FEBS Lett 1984; 167:37-41.
23. Penketh PG, Hodnick WF, Belcourt MF et al. Inhibition of DNA crosslinking by mitomycin C by peroxidase-mediated oxidation of mitomycin C hydroquinone. J Biol Chem 2001; 276:34445-34452.
24. Bartók M, Láng KL, Oxiranes. In: Patai S, ed. The chemistry of functional groups. Supplement E, Part 2, The chemistry of ether, Crown ethers, Hydroxyl groups and their sulphur analogues. Chichester: John Wiley Inc., 1980:609-673.
25. Degan P, Bonassi S, De Caterina M et al. In vivo accumulation of 8-hydroxy-2'-deoxyguanosine in DNA correlates with release of reactive oxygen species in Fanconi's anaemia families. Carcinogenesis 1995; 16:735-742.

26. Pagano G, Degan P, d'Ischia M et al. Gender- and age-related distinctions for the in vivo prooxidant state in Fanconi anaemia patients. Carcinogenesis 2004; 25:1899-1909.
27. Dufour C, Corcione A, Svahn J et al. TNF-α and IFN-γ are over expressed in the bone marrow of Fanconi anemia patients and TNF-α suppresses erythropoiesis in vitro. Blood 2003; 102:2053-2059.
28. Joenje H, Oostra AB. Clastogenicity of cyclophosphamide in Fanconi anemia lymphocytes without exogenous metabolic activation. Can Genet Cytogen1986; 22:339-345.
29. Joenje H, Arwert F, Eriksson AW et al. Oxygen-dependence of chromosomal aberrations in Fanconi's anaemia. Nature 1981; 290:142-143.
30. Raj AD, Heddle JA. The Effect of superoxide dismutase catalase, L cysteine on spontaneous and mitomycin C induced chromosomal breakage in Fanconi anemia and normal fibroblasts as measured by the micronucleus method. Mutat Res 1980; 78:59-66.
31. Reuter TY, Medhurst AL, Waisfisz Q et al. Yeast two-hybrid screens imply involvement of Fanconi anemia proteins in transcription regulation, cell signaling, oxidative metabolism, and cellular transport. Exp Cell Res 2003; 289:211-221.
32. Takeuchi T, Morimoto K. Increased formation of 8-hydroxydeoxyguanosine, an oxidative DNA damage, in lymphoblasts from Fanconi's anemia patients due to possible catalase deficiency. Carcinogenesis 1993; 14:1115-1120.
33. Zanier R, Briot D, Villard JA et al. Fanconi anemia C gene product regulates expression of genes involved in differentiation and inflammation. Oncogene 2004; 23:5004-5013.
34. Iyer VN, Szybalski W. Mitomycins and porphyromycin: Chemical mechanism of activation and cross-linking of DNA. Science 1964; 145:55-58.
35. Poot M, Gross O, Epe B et al. Cell cycle defect in connection with oxygen and iron sensitivity in Fanconi anemia lymphoblastoid cells. Exp Cell Res 1996; 222:262-268.
36. Bligh HFJ, Bartoszek A, Robson CN et al. Activation of mitomycin C by NADPH: Cytochrome P450 reductase. Cancer Res 1990; 50:7789-7792.
37. Pritsos CA, Sartorelli AC. Generation of reactive oxygen radicals through bioactivation of mitomycin antibiotic. Cancer Res 1986; 46:3528-3532.
38. Clarke AA, Philpott NJ, Gordon-Smith EC et al. The sensitivity of Fanconi anemia group C cells to apoptosis induced by mitomycin C is due to oxygen radical generation, not DNA crosslinking. Br J Haematol 1997; 96:240-247.
39. Korkina LG, Deeva IB, Iaccarino M et al. Redox dependent toxicity in diepoxybutane and mitomycin C in sea urchin embryogenesis. Carcinogenesis 2000; 21:213-220.
40. Ruppitsch W, Meisslitzer C, Hirsch-Kauffmann M et al. Overexpression of thioredoxin in Fanconi anemia fibroblasts prevents the cytotoxic and DNA damaging effect of mitomycin C and diepoxybutane. FEBS Lett 1998; 422:99-102.
41. Spanò M, Cordelli E, Leter G et al. Diepoxybutane cytotoxicity of mouse germ cells is enhanced by in vivo glutathione depletion. A flow cytometric approach. Mutat Res 1998; 397:37-43.
42. Vlachodimitropoulos D, Norppa H, Autio K et al. GSTT1-dependent induction of centromere-negative and -positive micronuclei by 1,2:3,4-diepoxybutane in cultured human lymphocytes. Mutagenesis 1997; 12:397-403.
43. Madle S. Evaluation of experimental parameters in an S9/human leukocyte SCE test with cyclophosphamide. Muatt Res 1981; 85:347-356.
44. Ghosh D, Das UB, Misra M. Protective role of alpha tocopherol -succinate (provitamin E) in cyclophosphamide induced testicular gametogenic and steroidogenic disorders: A correlative approach to oxidative stress. Free Radic Res 2002; 36:1209-1218.
45. De Martinis BS, Bianchi MD. Effect of vitamin C supplementation against cis-platin induced toxicity and oxidative DNA damage in rats. Pharmacol Res 2001; 44:317-320.
46. Schaaf GJ, Maas RF, de Groene EM et al. Management of oxidative stress by heme oxygenase-1 in cis-platin induced toxicity in renal tubular cells. Free Radic Res 2002; 36:835-843.
47. Goodbout JP, Pesavento J, Hartman ME et al. Methylglyoxal enhances cis-platin induced cytotoxicity by activating protein kinase C delta. J Biol Chem 2002; 277:2554-2561.
48. Waisfisz Q, Miyazato A, de Winter J et al. Analysis of baseline and cisplatin-inducible gene expression in Fanconi anemia cells using oligonucleotide-basedmicroarrays. BMC Blood Disorders 2002; 2:5.
49. Esposito F, Cuccovillo F, Russo L et al. A new $p21^{waf1/cip1}$ isoform is an early event of cell responce to oxidative stress. Cell Death Differ 1998; 5:940-945.
50. Zdzienicka MZ, Arwert F, Neuteboom I et al. The Chinese hamster V79 cell mutant V-h4 is phenotypically like Fanconi anemia cells. Somat Cell Mol Genet 1990; 16:575-581.
51. Decuyper J, Piette J, Van de Vorst A. Activated oxygen species produced by photoexcited furocoumarin derivatives. Arch Int Physiol Biochim 1983; 91:471-476.

52. Liu Z, Lu Y, Lebwohl M et al. PUVA (8-methoxypsoralen plus ultraviolet A) induces the formation of 8-hydroxy-2'-deoxyguanosine and DNA fragmentation in calf thymus DNA and human epidermoid carcinoma cells. Free Radic Biol Med 1999; 27:127-133.
53. d'Ischia M, Napolitano A, Prota G. Psoralen sensitise glutathione photooxidation in vitro. Biochim Biophys Acta 1989; 993:143-147.
54. Rousset S, Nocentini S, Rouillard D et al. Mitochondrial alterations in Fanconi anemia fibroblasts following ultraviolet A or psoralen photoactivation. Photochem Photobiol 2002; 75:159-166.
55. O'Brien T, Xu J, Patierno SR. Effects of glutathione on chromium induced DNA crosslinking and DNA polymerase arrest. Mol Cell Biochem 2001; 222:173-182.
56. Quievryn G, Goulart M, Messer J et al. Reduction of Cr (VI) by cysteine: Significance in human lymphocytes and formation of DNA damage in reaction with variable reduction rates. Mol Cell Biochem 2001; 222:107-118.
57. Izzotti A, Bagnasco M, Camoirano A et al. DNA fragmentation, DNA protein crosslinks, postlabeled nucleotide modifications and 8-hydroxy-2'-deoxyguanosine in the lung but not in liver of rats receiving intratracheal instillation of chromium (VI). Chemoprevention by oral N-acetlcysteine. Mutat Res 1998; 400:233-244.
58. Nguyen-nhu NT, Knoops B. Alkyl hydroperoxide 1 protects Saccharomyces cerevisiae against metal ion toxicity and glutathione depletion. Toxicol Lett 2002; 135:219-228.
59. Bagchi D, Bagchi M, Stohs SJ. Chromium (VI) induced oxidative stress, apoptotic cell death and modulation of p53 tumour suppressor gene. Mol Cell Biochem 2001; 222:149-158.
60. Tsou TC, Chen CL, Liu TY et al. Induction of 8-hydroxyguanosine in DNA by chromium (III) plus hydrogen peroxide and its prevention by scavengers. Carcinogenesis 1996; 17:103-108.
61. Park SJ, Ciccone SL, Beck BD et al. Oxidative stress/damage induces multimerization and interaction of Fanconi anemia proteins. J Biol Chem 2004; 279:30053-30059.
62. Morrell D, Chase CL, Kupper LL et al. Diabetes mellitus in ataxia-telangiectasia, Fanconi anemia, xeroderma pigmentosum, common variable immune deficiency, and severe combined immune deficiency families. Diabetes 1986; 35:143-147.
63. Dallapiccola B, Porfirio B, Mokini V et al. Effect of oxidants and anti-oxidants on chromosomal breakage in Fanconi anemia lymphocytes. Hum Genet 1985; 69:62-65.
64. Nagasawa H, Little JB. Suppression of cytotoxic effect of mitomycin-C by superoxide dismutase in Fanconi's anemia and dyskeratosis congenita fibroblasts. Carcinogenesis 1983; 4:795-798.
65. Saadatzadeh MR, Bijangi-Vishehsaraei K, Hong P et al. Oxidant hypersensitivity of Fanconi anemia type C deficient cells is dependent on a redox-regulated apoptotic pathway. J Biol Chem 2004; 279:16805-16812.
66. Emerit I, Levy A, Pagano G et al. Transferable clastogenic activity in plasma from patients with FA. Hum Genet 1995; 96:14-20.
67. Schulz JC, Shahidi NT. Tumor necrosis factor-α overproduction in Fanconi's anemia. Am J Hematol 1993; 42:196-201.
68. Pearl-Yafe M, Halperin D, Halevy A et al. An oxidative mechanism of interferon induced priming of the Fas pathway in Fanconi anemia cells. Biochem Pharmacol 2003; 65:833-842.
69. Kontou M, Adelfalk C, Ramirez MH et al. Overexpressed thioredoxin compensates Fanconi anemia related chromosomal instability. Oncogene 2002; 21:2406-2412.
70. Umegaki K, Sugisawa A, Shin SJ et al. Different onsets of oxidative damage to DNA and lipids in bone marrow and liver in rats given total body irradiation. Free Radic Biol Med 2001; 31:1066-1074.
71. Smith MT. Overview of benzene-induced aplastic anaemia. Eur J Haematol Suppl 1996; 60:107-110.
72. Memoli S, Napolitano A, d'Ischia M et al. Diffusible melanin-related metabolites are potent inhibitors of lipid peroxidation. Biochim Biophys Acta 1997; 1346:61-68.
73. Prota G. Melanins and Melanogenesis. New York: Academic Press, 1992.
74. Schallreuter KU, Lemke KR, Hill HZ et al. Thioredoxin reductase induction coincides with melanin biosynthesis in brown and black guinea pigs and in murine melanoma cells. J Invest Dermatol 1994; 103:820-824.
75. Schallreuter KU, Wood JM. Free radical reduction in the human epidermis. Free Radic Biol Med 1989; 6:519-532.
76. Wells PG, Kim PM, Laposa RR et al. Oxidative damage in chemical teratogenesis. Mutat Res 1997; 396:65-78.
77. Hansen JM, Harris KK, Philbert MA et al. Thalidomide modulates nuclear redox status and preferentially depletes glutathione in rabbit limb versus rat limb. J Pharmacol Exp Ther 2002; 300:768-776.
78. Blasiak J, Sikora A, Wozniak K et al. Genotoxicity of streptozotocin in normal and cancer cells and its modulation by free radical scavengers. Cell Biol Toxicol 2004; 20:83-96.

79. Tyrberg B, Anachkov KA, Dib SA et al. Islet expression of the DNA repair enzyme 8-oxoguanosine DNA glycosylase (Ogg1) in human type 2 diabetes. BMC Endocr Disord 2002; 2:2.
80. Ling G, Chadwick CA, Berne B et al. Epidermal p53 response and repair of thymine dimers in human skin after a single dose of ultraviolet radiation: Effects of photoprotection. Acta Derm Venereol 2001; 81:81-86.
81. Sheehan JM, Cragg N, Chadwick CA et al. Repeated ultraviolet exposure affords the same protection against DNA photodamage and erythema in human skin types II and IV but is associated with faster DNA repair in skin type IV. J Invest Dermatol 2002; 118:825-829.
82. Le Page F, Randrianarison V, Marot D et al. BRCA1 and BRCA2 are necessary for the transcription-coupled repair of the oxidative 8-oxoguanine lesion in human cells. Cancer Res 2000; 60:5548-5552.
83. Pichierri P, Rosselli F. The DNA crosslink-induced S-phase checkpoint depends on ATR-CHK1 and ATR-NBS1-FANCD2 pathways. EMBO J 2004; 23:1178-1187.
84. Howlett NG, Taniguchi T, Olson S et al. Biallelic inactivation of BRCA2 in Fanconi anemia. Science 2002; 297:606-609.
85. Das KC, Dashnamoorthy R. Hyperoxia activates the ATR-Chk1 pathway and phosphorylates p53 at multiple sites. Am J Physiol Lung Cell Mol Physiol 2004; 286:L87-97.

CHAPTER 10

Therapy for Fanconi Anemia

Madeleine Carreau*

Treatment of the hematological manifestation in Fanconi anemia is first supportive (transfusions) with attempts to stimulate hematopoiesis with either androgens, usually oxymetholone, or the hematopoietic growth factor granulocyte-colony stimulating factor (G-CSF), all of which are aimed at transiently improving peripheral blood counts. However, the long-term curative treatment of the hematological manifestation in Fanconi anemia patients is bone marrow (BM) or cord blood stem cell transplantation. The success rate for BM transplantation is fairly high with HLA-matched sibling donors but is, unfortunately, low with HLA-matched unrelated donors, making this procedure difficult for FA patients with no unaffected siblings. An alternative curative treatment for those patients with no sibling donors might be gene transfer into hematopoietic stem cells.

Androgens

Attempts to increase peripheral blood counts in FA patients are made, in some cases, using androgen therapy. The most common androgen used, oxymetholone, is a synthetic derivative of testosterone and has been approved by the US Food and Drug Administration (FDA) for the treatment of congenital and acquired anemia.[1] The recommended daily dose of oxymetholone is 1 to 5 mg/kg body weight per day in children and adults with anemias, the usual effective dose being between 1 and 2 mg/kg/day. Oxymetholone is well absorbed orally and has been shown to increase urinary erythropoietin (EPO) levels up to 5 fold.[2] Improvements in hemoglobin as well as increases in BM cellularity and in the number of neutrophils and platelets has been observed in aplastic anemia and Fanconi anemia cases with oxymetholone therapy.[3,4] However, several side effects are associated with the use of androgens such as masculinisation, acne, growth spurt followed by premature closing of epiphyses, hepatotoxicity, hepatic necrosis and tumorogenesis. Prolonged exposure to androgens in FA patients has been associated with hepatic function abnormalities and hepatic tumors.[5-7] Androgens are, in some cases, combined with corticosteroids such as prednisone to counterbalance the anabolic activity of androgens with the catabolic activity of corticosteroids believing that it may counteract the effect of androgen therapy on growth.[8,9]

Hematopoietic Growth Factors

Fanconi anemia cases unresponsive to androgens are generally treated with hematopoietic growth factors such as G-CSF. G-CSF has been shown to improve the hematological status of patients with acquired and inherited bone marrow failure.[10,11] In Fanconi anemia, only a few studies with hematopoietic growth factors have been reported.[12-15] FA patients were administered G-CSF at a daily dose of 2.5 to 7 ug/kg/day and most patients responded with an increase

*Madeleine Carreau—Department Pédiatrie, Université Laval, Unité de Recherche en Génétique Humaine et Moléculaire, CHUQ, Pavillon Saint-François d'Assise, 10, rue de l'Espinay, suite D0-711, Québec, Québec G1L 3L5 Canada. Email: madeleine.carreau@crsfa.ulaval.ca

Molecular Mechanisms of Fanconi Anemia, edited by Shamim I. Ahmad and Sandra H. Kirk. ©2006 Eurekah.com and Springer Science+Business Media.

in neutrophil counts. In some cases, CD34+ cells both in the peripheral blood and BM were also increased.[13] While Rackoff et al reported increased colony forming units-granulocyte-macrophage (CFU-GM) in FA patients treated with G-CSF for 10 months, the study by Scagni et al showed no effect on either burst forming units-erythrocytes (BFU-E) and CFU-GM following an 18 months G-CSF treatment. Treating FA with hematopoietic growth factors has raised some concerns regarding the potential of promoting the formation of leukemic clones or speeding the process of stem cell exhaustion. Since treatment of FA patients with G-CSF have been done on small cohorts and measured only in short-term periods, the long-term efficacy of such treatment and its impact on the progression of FA to myelodysplasia and AML have not been determined. Studies using the *Fancc* mouse model have shown that short-term use of cytokines, either G-CSF alone or in combination with EPO increased peripheral blood counts and delayed the onset of mitomycin C (MMC)-induced BM failure.[16] However, the study showed that long-term administration of hematopoietic growth factors increased sensitivity of *Fancc -/-* mice to MMC and dramatically decreased BM cellularity indicating that prolonged exposure may accelerate BM hypoplasia.

BM Transplants

Allogenic bone marrow or hematopoietic stem cell transplantation (BMT) is the only curative treatment for the hematological defect in FA. BMT for FA has been difficult in the context of designing a suitable conditioning regimen. Conditioning regimens often consist of radiation therapy combined with the DNA crosslinking agent cyclophosphamide (CY). CY generally used at a total dose of 200 mg/kg in conditioning regimens of aplastic anemia patients was shown to be toxic for Fanconi anemia patients leading to high transplanted-related mortality.[17] FA patients were also proven to be hypersensitive to irradiation showing increased radio-induced skin lesions.[18] Based on these observations, low dose CY (20 mg/kg over 4 days) and thoracoabdominal irradiation (TAI; 500 cGys) have been adopted as conditioning regimen of FA patients for BMT, which resulted in successful engraftment and low toxicity. Furthermore, antithymocyte globulin (ATG) has been added during the conditioning period and the posttransplant period and shown to improve the survival of FA patients.[19] Using this regimen, 151 FA patients transplanted between 1978 and 1994 with HLA-identical sibling donors and 48 with HLA-matched unrelated donors were reported in the International Bone Marrow Transplant Registry (IBMTR).[20] The 2-year survival was 66% for sibling donors and 29% with unrelated donors. Increased survival was associated with younger patient's age, higher pretransplant platelet counts, use of ATG, low-dose cyclophosphamide and reduced field irradiation for pretransplant conditioning regimen and cyclosporine for graft-versus-host-disease (GVHD) prophylaxis.[20] Thus, regimens consisting of low-dose CY (<100 mg/kg), such as the Paris and Cincinnati regimens,[19,20] gave better survival than regimens using more than 100 mg/kg of CY. However, other centers in Brazil and Saudi Arabia have reported that CY at a dose of 120 and 140 mg/kg with or without ATG but without irradiation gave long-term survival rates greater than 50%.[21,22] Differences between centers may reflect heterogeneity between FA patients in view of their complementation groups and specific mutations in the defective gene where some mutations may be more severe than others and thus, sensitivity to CY may vary from patient to patient as proposed by Ayas et al.[23] Nevertheless, reduced CY regimens (20 mg/kg) have been adopted by most centers including the Saudi Arabia centers[24] as the preferred conditioning regimen for patients with Fanconi anemia.

Unrelated Donors

In addition to difficulties with the conditioning regimen, transplants performed in FA with HLA-identical unrelated donors have been disappointing. While the success rate with HLA-matched sibling donors is between 60 and 70%, the survival using HLA-matched unrelated BMT is in the range of 29-34%.[20,25] A retrospective multicenter study was performed by the European Blood and Marrow Transplantation Group (EBMT) in collaboration with the European Fanconi Anemia Registry (EUFAR) in order to identify factors that were associated with poor outcome.[25] From January 1985 to June 1998, 69 FA patients were transplanted with BM cells from unrelated HLA-matched donors. The 3-year survival rate was determined at 33% and the probability of grade III-IV GVHD (graft versus host disease) was 34%. The day-100 transplant-related mortality was 39% where one third of the patients developed grade III-IV GVHD (acute GVHD was responsible for 13 out of 26 deaths). Association with worse outcome included cytomegalovirus positive serology, the use of androgens before transplant and female donors. A correlation was also established between the clinical phenotype and outcome, such as patients with congenital malformations had a 3-year survival of 14% compared to 44% for those with limited malformations. This low survival outcome was related to acute GVHD and graft failure. In addition, elevated serum alanine/aspartate transaminase values before the conditioning regimen, generally associated with pretransplant androgen therapy, were associated with a high day-100 mortality rate of 60% resulting mainly from acute GVHD where 9 out 11 patients with abnormal pretransplant transaminases died of GVHD. T-cell depletion, using either $CD34^+$ positive selection or negative selection based on ex-vivo antibody strategies was shown to be associated with a dramatic reduction in GVHD incidence with a 3 year overall survival of 44% compared to 27% with nonT-cell depleted grafts. Although GVHD is not the predominant lethal complication in the T-cell depleted group, primary and secondary graft failures appeared to be the major cause of complications post-transplant. No differences in survival were observed between the dose of CY used in preconditioning regimen (20 mg/kg at 34% survival compared to 40 mg/kg at 31% survival) or the type of irradiation (total body irradiation with 35% survival versus thoracoabdominal irradiation with 33% survival).

Currently the EBMT Group are using a modified conditioning regimen for unrelated HLA-matched BMT for FA patients consisting of a higher dose of CY (10 mg/kg/day, days -6, -5, -4, -3, total dose of 40 mg/kg) with a single dose of 4.5 Gy (dose rate 26 cGy/min) total-body irradiation and ATG (12 mg/kg, days -6 to -1, six doses) followed by T-cell depletion using $CD34^+$ cell selection methods. This new protocol has been promising showing 9 out of 11 FA patients alive with good engraftment and minimal GVHD at the time of the report.[26]

Cord Blood

For patients with no available related donor, cord blood or placental blood provides an alternative source of hematopoietic stem cells. This source of hematopoietic cells also offers several advantages such as relative ease to obtain, small risk of transmitting infections (CMV or EBV) and low risk of GVHD due to immunological immaturity of cord blood cells. This may also permit more HLA-mismatch between donor and recipient. The first successful transplant for a patient with Fanconi anemia using umbilical cord blood was done in 1988 using a sibling HLA-matched donor.[27] Since then, cord blood banks have been developed world-wide for the collection, testing and cryopreserving of cord blood hematopoietic cells from both related and unrelated donors.[28-30]

In 1992, a Placental Blood Program at the New York Blood Center has been established in order to make cord blood available to transplantation centers.[31] Since 1992, this program has provided placental blood to 98 transplantation centers for a total of 562 transplants all with unrelated donor cells for the treatment of various hematological disorders.[31] Of these 562 recipients, 35 had been diagnosed with Fanconi anemia. A report from this program indicated that placental cord blood transplants regularly engrafted, caused low rate GVHD and produced survival rates (100 days survival of 46%) similar to BMT from unrelated donors. However, patients with Fanconi anemia reported in this study, showed poor engraftment. In Europe, 143 cord-blood transplantations performed between 1988 and 1996 have been reported.[32] Of these 143 recipients (16 FA patients), 65 (8 FA patients) were transplanted with unrelated donor cord blood cells. The one-year survival for recipients transplanted with cord blood from unrelated donors was 29%. Most patients died of complications including GVHD, interstitial pneumonitis, acute respiratory distress syndrome, cardiac failure, veno-occlusive liver disease, rejection, infections and hemorrhage.[32]

Fludarabine Based Conditioning Regimen

To overcome the risk of organ toxicity or GVHD while ensuring high levels of engraftment in FA patients with unrelated donors, some forms of T-cell depletion was used and showed to prevent GVHD without the morbidity of methotrexate or cyclosporine.[25] However, T-cell depletion in unrelated donor transplant was associated with higher incidence of graft rejection. Thus, low-intensity, nonmyeloablative but highly immunosuppressive regimens consisting of fludarabine have been tested for Fanconi anemia patients. Fludarabine monophosphate is a purine analogue relatively nontoxic that causes severe T-cell depletion by inhibiting adenosine deaminase.[33,34] This immunosuppressive agent has been proven effective as a conditioning agent for chronic lymphocytic leukemia patients. The first FA patient who underwent BMT using fludarabine in combination with ATG and cyclophosphamide as a preparative regimen was reported in 1997.[35] This patient had thrombocytopenia with leukemic transformation before undergoing BMT. Engraftment was rapid with no transplant-related complications or GVHD. After 10 months post-BMT, the patient had a 100% chimerism and was in excellent clinical condition. This novel fludarabine-based preparative regimen without irradiation was used to treat successfully other FA patients with either related-mismatched donor stem cells or HLA-mismatched unrelated donors.[36-38] In all cases, engraftment was normal and sustained. The regimen was well tolerated with very mild toxicity and no major transplant-related complications were observed.

The fludarabine-based preparative regimen was also used in combination with irradiation in some cases. For instance, one FA patient presenting a life-threatening aplastic anemia with no matched sibling donor underwent a haploidentical peripheral blood stem cell transplant using the Gluckman protocol (low CY, reduced TAI and ATG).[39] However, graft rejection occurred and this patient underwent a second transplant, this time, following a 5 day fludarabine treatment which led to successful engraftment. Similarly, one FA patient was reported to achieve successful engraftment following a second CD34$^+$ cell dose from the same donor after fludarabine and ATG treatment.[40] Fludarabine was also used in combination with low-dose total body irradiation (TBI) without CY.[41] The regimen was well tolerated with minimal complications during the transplant period with gradual engraftment and no GVHD.

BMT Complications

Opportunistic infections such as cytomegalovirus (CMV) and fungal infections have now become a major concern of complications during BMT. The use of ATG before and after BMT has helped target the cells responsible for graft rejection and graft-versus-host-disease (GVHD) but at the same time has increased the risk of opportunistic infections in the post-transplant period. While the Cincinnati group[19] demonstrated that use of ATG pre and post-transplant was associated with good engraftment and low GVHD, Ayas et al reported that ATG was associated with higher incidence of life-threatening CMV and fungal infections.[24] Although the Cincinnati group reported no cases of CMV infections, half of their patients/recipients were CMV seronegative. Based on these studies, the Saudi Arabia center has now included prophylactic anti-fungal agents such as fluconazole on all FA patients undergoing BMT. However, studies using lower doses of ATG are also being considered.

Another major concern of BMT in FA patients is the high incidence of secondary tumors after transplant. The probability of developing malignant tumors in FA patients is very high due to the chromosomal instability associated with the disease. FA patients are at a higher risk of developing malignancies, the most common being hematological in nature, but FA patients are also at increased risk of developing nonhematological (solid) tumors, particularly squamous cell carcinomas.[42-44] Alkylating agents with or without irradiation used as conditioning regimens in association with the disease susceptibility to cancer are all contributing factors to tumor formation post-transplant. Most solid tumors observed in FA patients post-transplant are squamous cell carcinomas of the head and neck.[45,46] Head and neck squamous cell carcinoma is also the most frequent nonhematological cancer observed in FA (24% of all nonhematological cancer). A joint analysis between the Seattle and the Paris transplant groups has identified that the most significant risk factor for tumor development in Fanconi anemia patients was acute GVHD followed by the administration of immunosuppressive agents such as azathioprine for the treatment of chronic GVHD.[45] No lymphoproliferative malignancies were observed post-transplant in FA patients, which is consistent with the fact that transplantation provides hematological correction without correction to other tissues. The use of irradiation as part of the conditioning regimen has also been associated with a significant risk for secondary tumors in nonFanconi aplastic anemia patients.[45] In view of the hypersensitivity in FA patients to radiation therapy[18] and patient's cells to DNA damaging agents,[47] the risk of developing secondary tumors could also be higher in FA patients with irradiation as part of the conditioning regimen. However, since FA patients who did not receive irradiation as part of their conditioning regimen also developed late cancers, radiation therapy is not the only risk factor contributing to secondary tumors in FA.[22] In addition, the use of CY, a DNA damaging agent, in conditioning regimen for FA patients may also contribute, to some extent, to the formation of secondary tumors since tissues other than bone marrow have not been corrected from the DNA repair defect associated with the disease.

The ideal conditioning regimen and post-transplant immunosuppression for FA patients has yet to be determined. Investigators are still searching for the best preparative regimen that will reduce the risk of toxicities while providing high levels of engraftment. Taken as a whole, recent studies suggest that highly immunosuppresive regimen consisting of fludarabine, low-dose CY and ATG with or without radiation therapy can provide, for FA patients with unrelated donors, stable long-lasting engraftment with only mild toxicity.

Gene Therapy

The only long-term treatment for FA has been transplantation of bone marrow or umbilical cord hematopoietic cells. The success rate for BM transplantation is fairly high with HLA-matched siblings but is, unfortunately, low with HLA-matched unrelated donors, making this procedure difficult for FA patients with no unaffected siblings. An alternative curative treatment for those patients with no sibling donors might be gene transfer into hematopoietic stem cells. Stem and progenitor cells can easily be harvested from the bone marrow or peripheral blood and transduced ex vivo using viral vectors as a delivery system. In view of their self-renewal capacity, corrected stem cells, in theory, could replenish the hematopoietic compartment and sustain long-term hematopoiesis.

Recombinant viral vectors have been engineered as delivery systems for the transfer of genetic material in a target cell. Retroviral vectors derived from oncoretroviruses such as the murine leukemia virus (MLV) have been widely used in gene transfer experiments and were shown to have the advantage of integrating into the host genome. However, they do not efficiently infect nondividing cells such as human hematopoietic stem cells because the preintegration complex is unable to traverse the intact nuclear membrane.[48] Since hematopoietic stem cells are generally quiescent, growth factors have been used to stimulate cells, however, exposure to cytokines often lead to differentiation and loss of homing abilities of stem cells and in turn reduce their long-term repopulating potential.[49-51] Adenoviruses and adeno-associated viruses (AAV) are DNA viruses that can transduce dividing and nondividing cells. However, adenoviruses do not integrate into the host genome and expression of the transgene lasts only a short time, which is not ideal for long-term corrective effect as needed in FA. Adenoviral and AAV vectors were also shown to be very immunogenic and transduced cells are rapidly cleared from the body.[52,53] Other limitations with AAV vectors are transgene size, 3 to 4 kb, and the need for helper virus (usually adenovirus or herpes simplex virus) for its replication which makes purification procedure laborious in order to separate the targeting vector from helper viruses.[54,55] Recent advances in human immunodeficiency virus (HIV) research have paved the way for use of lentiviruses for gene transfer studies into nondividing cells[56-58] Lentiviruses also belong to the retrovirus family, but they have the ability to infect nondividing as well as dividing cells. Lentivirus HIV-1 and HIV-2 based vectors have now been engineered to reduce the risks of recombination and have been shown to efficiently and stably transduce nondividing cells without immune reaction or generation of replication competent virus.[59-64]

Retroviral, AAV and lentiviral vectors have been used to deliver normal copies of *FANC* genes into FA deficient cell lines.[65-69] These vectors were shown to be successful in vitro assays showing phenotypic correction of the MMC hypersensitivity in FA cells. In addition, transduction of mobilized peripheral blood CD34$^+$ cells isolated form a FA group C patient showed functional complementation as measured by improved colony formation following transduction with the *FANCC* gene.[65,66,70] Similar results were obtained following transduction of FA group A hematopoietic progenitors with a retroviral vector encoding the *FANCA* gene showing improved colony growth evaluated by both size and numbers.[68]

In view of the successful correction of the FA cellular phenotype upon transduction using various viral vectors, gene delivery into hematopoietic cells has been evaluated in vivo using animal models. In FA, three mouse models have been generated by disruption the mouse respective *Fanc* locus, *Fanca*, *Fancc* and *Fancg*.[71-74] Cells obtained from FA mutant mice were shown to be hypersensitive to DNA crosslinking agents and to have abnormal G_2/M progression of the cell cycle similar to that seen in FA patient cells.[72,75,76] Also, hematopoietic progenitor cells from *Fancc* -/- mice were shown to be hypersensitive to many cytokines including TNFα, IFN-γ and MIP-1α showing reduced colony growth and increased apoptosis.[73,77-79] In addition to the cellular phenotype, bone marrow failure similar to that observed in FA patients was shown in *Fancc* -/- mice after treatment with the DNA damaging agent mitomycin C.[80] These Fanc-deficient mice have enable investigators to test the efficacy of various viral vectors in complementing the cellular and in vivo phenotype. Long-term repopulating hematopoietic progenitor cells obtained from *Fanca* -/- mice have been transduced with the human *FANCA* gene using retroviral vectors.[81] Results showed that the *FANCA* transgene corrected the MMC hypersensitivity and impaired ex vivo expansion ability of *Fanca* -/- hematopoietic progenitor cells. Furthermore, successful complementation of the in vivo hypersensitivity to MMC of *Fancc* -/- mice has been obtained with total BM cells transduced with either retroviral or lentiviral vectors encoding the human *FANCC* gene.[82,83]

The potential for successful gene therapy in FA has been supported by a natural phenomenon called somatic mosaicism, observed in some FA patient lymphocytes where populations of lymphocytes were no longer sensitive to DNA crosslinking agents.[84]

This in vivo selective advantage has also been reproduced in the FA group C mouse model (*Fancc* -/-) by transplantation of normal wild-type hematopoietic cells.[85] These findings imply that the reverted cell has had a selective advantage over the nonreverted ones and suggest that efficient gene transfer in only a few pluripotent hematopoietic cells would be enough to restore normal hematopoiesis in FA patients.

A clinical trial for 3 FA group C patients is in progress where G-CSF-mobilized BM progenitors have been transduced ex vivo with a retroviral based vector encoding the *FANCC* gene.[86] Because of retroviral vectors inefficiency to transduced hematopoietic stem cells, this study included four cycles of mobilization, collection, transduction and infusion in order to increase the number of corrected cells. Prior to infusion, presence of the *FANCC* transgene in transduced CD34-enriched progenitor cells has been demonstrated. Following infusion, FANCC was also present in peripheral blood and BM cells. Functionality of the transgene has been demonstrated in vitro by clonogenic assays with or without MMC and in vivo by increased BM cellularity. In addition, one patient that had been given radiation therapy for a malignancy showed *FANCC* transgene expression in peripheral blood and BM only after recovery from radiation-induced aplasia suggesting that *FANCC* transduced cells had had a selective growth advantage.[86] However, despite the growth advantage of transduced cells, there has been no long-term evidence of in vivo amplification of a corrected hematopoietic stem cell in the 3 patients undergoing gene therapy treatment.

One of the problems with the current gene therapy protocol is the low efficiency of hematopoietic stem cell transduction. Since hematopoietic stem cells do not replicate, other vectors such as lentiviral-based vectors might have a better chance of success. The amount of stem cells found in BM from FA patients may be reduced due to BM aplasia and may thus be a limiting factor for gene therapy. Preliminary results using the SCID mouse xenotransplant model, showed that BM from FA patients contained too few stem cells to enable reconstitution of hematopoiesis.[87] Another major issue that can limit successful treatment by gene transfer is insertional mutagenesis that could trigger leukemia. Recently, two severe combined immunodeficiency disease (SCID) patients out of 11 patients treated by gene therapy were diagnosed with leukemia.[88] Cells from both patients showed the same molecular event where the transgene had been inserted at the *LMO2* gene locus and was associated with aberrant *LMO2* gene expression. Aberrant expression of LMO2 caused by chromosomal translocation has been reported in acute lymphoblastic leukemia.[89] This finding prompted the United States Food and Drug Administration to temporary halt similar gene therapy trials using retroviral vectors in blood stem cells.[90] Since FA patients have higher risks of developing leukemia and are subjected to many chromosomal translocations, corrected cells may be predisposed to malignancy and insertional mutagenesis may trigger leukemia post-gene therapy.

Gene therapy is still in its infancy and many aspects need to be resolved before it is widely used as a form of treatment. However, for patients with no alternative treatments, for instance, FA patients with no HLA-matched BM donors, gene transfer may still provide a cure for the hematopoietic defect. Assessing the risk of gene therapy in FA may thus require more preclinical investigation and basic research for the development of safer transfer vectors and determination of potential insertional sites.

Prospects for Therapy

Introduction of bioactive FA proteins directly into FA-deficient cells has been explored as a potential corrective therapy. Although protein replacement therapy has received less attention than gene therapy, specifically for FA, in vitro studies have provided promising results. Chimeric proteins consisting of a FA protein in fusion to a cell surface receptor (either IL-3 or CD33) have been designed to target cells expressing these specific receptors.[91,92] Upon binding to the receptor, the chimeric protein is internalized and can function normally as shown by complementation of the MMC sensitivity in FA deficient-cells. These preliminary results, however, need to be supported with testing in hematopoietic cells as well as in an in vivo setting, for instance using *Fanc*-deficient mice. Unlike gene therapy, protein replacement does not involve any risk of insertional mutagenesis, however, many questions remain to be answered, such as, is the protein half-life (60 minutes for FANCC and 160 minutes for FANCF) long enough for in vivo function? What would be the ideal method of systemic distribution? Will the chimeric protein need to be targeted to hematopoietic stem cells or would any progenitor cell suffice for correction of the hematopoieic defect. Nevertheless, the transfer of bioactive proteins could provide an interesting adjunctive therapy for FA until a definitive treatment of choice can be made.

Conclusion

For now, the treatment of choice for FA patients remains BMT with a HLA-identical sibling donor. Improved preconditioning regimen and immunosuppresive therapy post-transplant has increased the success rate of BMT for FA patients, although secondary tumors post-transplant remains a major concern. Results of unrelated matched transplants and family related mismatched transplants have improved over the past few years with the use of T-cell depletion and fludarabine therapy. However, the success rate is still low and other forms of therapy such as gene transfer, or eventually protein transfer, may be a possible alternative.

References

1. Pavlatos AM, Fultz O, Monberg MJ et al. Review of oxymetholone: A 17alpha-alkylated anabolic-androgenic steroid. Clin Ther 2001; 23(6):789-801; discussion 771.
2. Alexanian R, Nadell J, Alfrey C. Oxymetholone treatment for the anemia of bone marrow failure. Blood 1972; 40(3):353-365.
3. Sanchez-Medal L, Gomez-Leal A, Duarte L et al. Anabolic androgenic steroids in the treatment of acquired aplastic anemia. Blood 1969; 34(3):283-300.
4. Claustres M, Margueritte G, Sultan C. In vitro CFU-E and BFU-E responses to androgen in bone marrow from children with primary hypoproliferative anaemia: A possible therapeutic assay. Eur J Pediatr 1986; 144(5):467-471.
5. Touraine RL, Bertrand Y, Foray P et al. Hepatic tumours during androgen therapy in Fanconi anaemia. Eur J Pediatr 1993; 152(8):691-693.
6. Schmidt E, Deeg HJ, Storb R. Regression of androgen-related hepatic tumors in patients with Fanconi's anemia following marrow transplantation. Transplantation 1984; 37(5):452-455.
7. Shapiro P, Ikeda RM, Ruebner BH et al. Multiple hepatic tumors and peliosis hepatis in Fanconi's anemia treated with androgens. Am J Dis Child 1977; 131(10):1104-1106.
8. Pedersen FK, Hertz H, Lundsteen C et al. Indication of primary immune deficiency in Fanconi's anemia. Acta Paediatr Scand 1977; 66(6):745-751.
9. Bacigalupo A, Chaple M, Hows J et al. Treatment of aplastic anaemia (AA) with antilymphocyte globulin (ALG) and methylprednisolone (MPred) with or without androgens: A randomized trial from the EBMT SAA working party. Br J Haematol 1993; 83(1):145-151.
10. Antin JH, Smith BR, Holmes W et al. Phase I/II study of recombinant human granulocyte-macrophage colony-stimulating factor in aplastic anemia and myelodysplastic syndrome. Blood 1988; 72(2):705-713.
11. Guinan EC, Sieff CA, Oette DH et al. A phase I/II trial of recombinant granulocyte-macrophage colony-stimulating factor for children with aplastic anemia. Blood 1990; 76(6):1077-1082.
12. Scagni P, Saracco P, Timeus F et al. Use of recombinant granulocyte colony-stimulating factor in Fanconi's anemia. Haematologica 1998; 83(5):432-437.
13. Rackoff WR, Orazi A, Robinson CA et al. Prolonged administration of granulocyte colony-stimulating factor (filgrastim) to patients with Fanconi anemia: A pilot study. Blood 1996; 88(5):1588-1593.
14. Kemahli S, Canatan D, Uysal Z et al. GM-CSF in the treatment of Fanconi's anaemia. Br J Haematol 1994; 87(4):871-872.
15. Guinan EC, Lopez KD, Huhn RD et al. Evaluation of granulocyte-macrophage colony-stimulating factor for treatment of pancytopenia in children with fanconi anemia. J Pediatr 1994; 124(1):144-150.
16. Carreau M, Liu L, Gan OI et al. Short-term granulocyte colony-stimulating factor and erythropoietin treatment enhances hematopoiesis and survival in the mitomycin C- conditioned Fancc(-/-) mouse model, while long-term treatment is ineffective. Blood 2002; 100(4):1499-1501.
17. Gluckman E, Devergie A, Schaison G et al. Bone marrow transplantation in Fanconi anaemia. Br J Haematol 1980; 45(4):557-564.
18. Gluckman E, Devergie A, Dutreix J. Radiosensitivity in Fanconi anaemia: Application to the conditioning regimen for bone marrow transplantation. Br J Haematol 1983; 54(3):431-440.
19. Kohli-Kumar M, Morris C, DeLaat C et al. Bone marrow transplantation in Fanconi anemia using matched sibling donors. Blood 1994; 84(6):2050-2054.
20. Gluckman E, Auerbach AD, Horowitz MM et al. Bone marrow transplantation for Fanconi anemia. Blood 1995; 86(7):2856-2862.
21. Zanis-Neto J, Ribeiro RC, Medeiros C et al. Bone marrow transplantation for patients with Fanconi anemia: A study of 24 cases from a single institution. Bone Marrow Transplant 1995; 15(2):293-298.
22. Flowers ME, Zanis J, Pasquini R et al. Marrow transplantation for Fanconi anaemia: Conditioning with reduced doses of cyclophosphamide without radiation. Br J Haematol 1996; 92(3):699-706.
23. Ayas M, Mustafa MM. Results of allogeneic BMT in 16 patients with Fanconi's anemia. Bone Marrow Transplant 2000; 25(12):1321-1322.
24. Ayas M, Solh H, Mustafa MM et al. Bone marrow transplantation from matched siblings in patients with fanconi anemia utilizing low-dose cyclophosphamide, thoracoabdominal radiation and antithymocyte globulin. Bone Marrow Transplant 2001; 27(2):139-143.
25. Guardiola P, Pasquini R, Dokal I et al. Outcome of 69 allogeneic stem cell transplantations for Fanconi anemia using HLA-matched unrelated donors: A study on behalf of the European Group for Blood and Marrow Transplantation. Blood 2000; 95(2):422-429.
26. Gluckman E, Socié G, Guardiaola P. Treatment of Fanconi's anemia. In: Schrezenmeier H, Bacigalupo A, eds. Aplastic Anemia: Pathophysiology and treatment. Cambridge, UK: Cambridge University Press, 2000:391.

27. Gluckman E, Broxmeyer HA, Auerbach AD et al. Hematopoietic reconstitution in a patient with Fanconi's anemia by means of umbilical-cord blood from an HLA-identical sibling. New England Journal of Medicine 1989; 321(17):1174-1178.
28. Rubinstein P, Dobrila L, Rosenfield RE et al. Processing and cryopreservation of placental/umbilical cord blood for unrelated bone marrow reconstitution. Proc Natl Acad Sci USA 1995; 92(22):10119-10122.
29. Silberstein LE, Jefferies LC. Placental-blood banking—a new frontier in transfusion medicine. N Engl J Med 1996; 335(3):199-201.
30. Wagner JE, Rosenthal J, Sweetman R et al. Successful transplantation of HLA-matched and HLA-mismatched umbilical cord blood from unrelated donors: Analysis of engraftment and acute graft-versus-host disease. Blood 1996; 88(3):795-802.
31. Rubinstein P, Carrier C, Scaradavou A et al. Outcomes among 562 recipients of placental-blood transplants from unrelated donors. N Engl J Med 1998; 339(22):1565-1577.
32. Gluckman E, Rocha V, Boyer-Chammard A et al. Outcome of cord-blood transplantation from related and unrelated donors. Eurocord transplant group and the european blood and marrow transplantation group. N Engl J Med 1997; 337(6):373-381.
33. Huang P, Chubb S, Plunkett W. Termination of DNA synthesis by 9-beta-D-arabinofuranosyl-2-fluoroadenine. A mechanism for cytotoxicity. J Biol Chem 1990; 265(27):16617-16625.
34. Plunkett W, Huang P, Gandhi V. Metabolism and action of fludarabine phosphate. Semin Oncol 1990; 17(5 Suppl 8):3-17.
35. Kapelushnik J, Or R, Slavin S et al. A fludarabine-based protocol for bone marrow transplantation in Fanconi's anemia. Bone Marrow Transplant 1997; 20(12):1109-1110.
36. Aker M, Varadi G, Slavin S et al. Fludarabine-based protocol for human umbilical cord blood transplantation in children with Fanconi anemia. J Pediatr Hematol Oncol 1999; 21(3):237-239.
37. Boulad F, Gillio A, Small TN et al. Stem cell transplantation for the treatment of Fanconi anaemia using a fludarabine-based cytoreductive regimen and T-cell-depleted related HLA- mismatched peripheral blood stem cell grafts. Br J Haematol 2000; 111(4):1153-1157.
38. Rossi G, Giorgiani G, Comoli P et al. Successful T-cell-depleted, related haploidentical peripheral blood stem cell transplantation in a patient with Fanconi anaemia using a fludarabine-based preparative regimen without radiation. Bone Marrow Transplant 2003; 31(6):437-440.
39. Elhasid R, Ben Arush MW, Katz T et al. Successful haploidentical bone marrow transplantation in Fanconi anemia. Bone Marrow Transplant 2000; 26(11):1221-1223.
40. Ortin M, Raj R, Kinning E et al. Partially matched related donor peripheral blood progenitor cell transplantation in paediatric patients adding fludarabine and anti-lymphocyte gamma-globulin. Bone Marrow Transplant 2002; 30(6):359-366.
41. de Medeiros CR, Silva LM, Pasquini R. Unrelated cord blood transplantation in a Fanconi anemia patient using fludarabine-based conditioning. Bone Marrow Transplant 2001; 28(1):110-112.
42. Alter BP. Cancer in Fanconi anemia, 1927-2001. Cancer 2003; 97(2):425-440.
43. Kutler DI, Singh B, Satagopan J et al. A 20-year perspective on the International Fanconi Anemia Registry (IFAR). Blood 2003; 101(4):1249-1256.
44. Kutler DI, Auerbach AD, Satagopan J et al. High incidence of head and neck squamous cell carcinoma in patients with Fanconi anemia. Arch Otolaryngol Head Neck Surg 2003; 129(1):106-112.
45. Deeg HJ, Socie G, Schoch G et al. Malignancies after marrow transplantation for aplastic anemia and fanconi anemia: A joint Seattle and Paris analysis of results in 700 patients. Blood 1996; 87(1):386-392.
46. Socie G, Henry-Amar M, Cosset JM et al. Increased incidence of solid malignant tumors after bone marrow transplantation for severe aplastic anemia [see comments]. Blood 1991; 78(2):277-279.
47. Carreau M, Alon N, Bosnoyan-Collins L et al. Drug sensitivity spectra in Fanconi anemia lymphoblastoid cell lines of defined complementation groups. Mutat Res 1999; 435(1):103-109.
48. Roe T, Reynolds TC, Yu G et al. Integration of murine leukemia virus DNA depends on mitosis. EMBO J 1993; 12(5):2099-2108.
49. Bhatia M, Bonnet D, Kapp U et al. Quantitative analysis reveals expansion of human hematopoietic repopulating cells after short-term ex vivo culture. J Exp Med 1997; 186(4):619-624.
50. Tisdale JF, Hanazono Y, Sellers SE et al. Ex vivo expansion of genetically marked rhesus peripheral blood progenitor cells results in diminished long-term repopulating ability. Blood 1998; 92(4):1131-1141.
51. Takatoku M, Sellers S, Agricola BA et al. Avoidance of stimulation improves engraftment of cultured and retrovirally transduced hematopoietic cells in primates. J Clin Invest 2001; 108(3):447-455.
52. Dai Y, Schwarz EM, Gu D et al. Cellular and humoral immune responses to adenoviral vectors containing factor IX gene: Tolerization of factor IX and vector antigens allows for long-term expression. Proc Natl Acad Sci USA 1995; 92(5):1401-1405.

53. Yang Y, Haecker SE, Su Q et al. Immunology of gene therapy with adenoviral vectors in mouse skeletal muscle. Hum Mol Genet 1996; 5(11):1703-1712.
54. Grimm D, Kern A, Rittner K et al. Novel tools for production and purification of recombinant adenoassociated virus vectors. Hum Gene Ther 1998; 9(18):2745-2760.
55. Wang XS, Khuntirat B, Qing K et al. Characterization of wild-type adeno-associated virus type 2-like particles generated during recombinant viral vector production and strategies for their elimination. J Virol 1998; 72(7):5472-5480.
56. Naldini L, Blomer U, Gallay P et al. In vivo gene delivery and stable transduction of nondividing cells by a lentiviral vector. Science 1996; 272(5259):263-267.
57. Naldini L. Lentiviruses as gene transfer agents for delivery to nondividing cells. Curr Opin Biotechnol 1998; 9(5):457-463.
58. Verma IM, Somia N. Gene therapy—promises, problems and prospects. Nature 1997; 389(6648):239-242.
59. Luther-Wyrsch A, Costello E, Thali M et al. Stable transduction with lentiviral vectors and amplification of immature hematopoietic progenitors from cord blood of preterm human fetuses. Hum Gene Ther 2001; 12(4):377-389.
60. Barrette S, Douglas JL, Seidel NE et al. Lentivirus-based vectors transduce mouse hematopoietic stem cells with similar efficiency to moloney murine leukemia virus-based vectors. Blood 2000; 96(10):3385-3391.
61. Guenechea G, Gan OI, Inamitsu T et al. Transduction of human CD34+ CD38- bone marrow and cord blood-derived SCID-repopulating cells with third-generation lentiviral vectors. Mol Ther 2000; 1(6):566-573.
62. Miyoshi H, Smith KA, Mosier DE et al. Transduction of human CD34+ cells that mediate long-term engraftment of NOD/SCID mice by HIV vectors. Science 1999; 283(5402):682-686.
63. Sutton RE, Wu HT, Rigg R et al. Human immunodeficiency virus type 1 vectors efficiently transduce human hematopoietic stem cells. J Virol 1998; 72(7):5781-5788.
64. Uchida N, Sutton RE, Friera AM et al. HIV, but not murine leukemia virus, vectors mediate high efficiency gene transfer into freshly isolated G0/G1 human hematopoietic stem cells. Proc Natl Acad Sci USA 1998; 95(20):11939-11944.
65. Walsh CE, Nienhuis AW, Samulski RJ et al. Phenotypic correction of Fanconi anemia in human hematopoietic cells with a recombinant adeno-associated virus vector. J Clin Invest 1994; 94(4):1440-1448.
66. Walsh CE, Grompe M, Vanin E et al. A functionally active retrovirus vector for gene therapy in Fanconi anemia group C. Blood 1994; 84(2):453-459.
67. Machl AW, Planitzer S, Kubbies M. A novel, membrane receptor-based retroviral vector for Fanconi anemia group C gene therapy. Gene Ther 1997; 4(4):339-345.
68. Fu KL, Foe JR, Joenje H et al. Functional correction of Fanconi anemia group A hematopoietic cells by retroviral gene transfer. Blood 1997; 90(9):3296-3303.
69. Yamada K, Olsen JC, Patel M et al. Functional correction of fanconi anemia group C hematopoietic cells by the use of a novel lentiviral vector. Mol Ther 2001; 3(4):485-490.
70. Walsh CE, Mann MM, Emmons RV et al. Transduction of CD34-enriched human peripheral and umbilical cord blood progenitors using a retroviral vector with the Fanconi anemia group C gene. J Investig Med 1995; 43(4):379-385.
71. Chen M, Tomkins DJ, Auerbach W et al. Inactivation of Fac in mice produces inducible chromosomal instability and reduced fertility reminiscent of Fanconi anaemia. Nat Genet 1996; 12(4):448-451.
72. Cheng NC, van de Vrugt HJ, van der Valk MA et al. Mice with a targeted disruption of the Fanconi anemia homolog Fanca. Hum Mol Genet 2000; 9(12):1805-1811.
73. Whitney MA, Royle G, Low MJ et al. Germ cell defects and hematopoietic hypersensitivity to gamma- interferon in mice with a targeted disruption of the Fanconi anemia C gene. Blood 1996; 88(1):49-58.
74. Yang Y, Kuang Y, De Oca RM et al. Targeted disruption of the murine Fanconi anemia gene, Fancg/Xrcc9. Blood 2001; 98(12):3435-3440.
75. Tomkins DJ, Care M, Carreau M et al. Development and characterization of immortalized fibroblastoid cell lines from an FA(C) mouse model. Mutat Res 1998; 408(1):27-35.
76. Otsuki T, Wang J, Demuth I et al. Assessment of mitomycin C sensitivity in Fanconi anemia complementation group C gene (Fac) knock-out mouse cells. Int J Hematol 1998; 67(3):243-248.
77. Haneline LS, Broxmeyer HE, Cooper S et al. Multiple inhibitory cytokines induce deregulated progenitor growth and apoptosis in hematopoietic cells from Fac-/- mice. Blood 1998; 91(11):4092-4098.

78. Rathbun RK, Christianson TA, Faulkner GR et al. Interferon-gamma-induced apoptotic responses of Fanconi anemia group C hematopoietic progenitor cells involve caspase 8-dependent activation of caspase 3 family members. Blood 2000; 96(13):4204-4211.
79. Rathbun RK, Faulkner GR, Ostroski MH et al. Inactivation of the Fanconi anemia group C gene augments interferon- gamma-induced apoptotic responses in hematopoietic cells. Blood 1997; 90(3):974-985.
80. Carreau M, Gan OI, Liu L et al. Bone marrow failure in the Fanconi anemia group C mouse model after DNA damage. Blood 1998; 91(8):2737-2744.
81. Rio P, Segovia JC, Hanenberg H et al. In vitro phenotypic correction of hematopoietic progenitors from Fanconi anemia group A knockout mice. Blood 2002; 100(6):2032-2039.
82. Gush KA, Fu KL, Grompe M et al. Phenotypic correction of Fanconi anemia group C knockout mice. Blood 2000; 95(2):700-704.
83. Galimi F, Noll M, Kanazawa Y et al. Gene therapy of Fanconi anemia: Preclinical efficacy using lentiviral vectors. Blood 2002; 100(8):2732-2736.
84. Lo Ten Foe JR, Kwee ML, Rooimans MA et al. Somatic mosaicism in Fanconi anemia: Molecular basis and clinical significance. Eur J Hum Genet 1997; 5(3):137-148.
85. Battaile KP, Bateman RL, Mortimer D et al. In vivo selection of wild-type hematopoietic stem cells in a murine model of Fanconi anemia. Blood 1999; 94(6):2151-2158.
86. Liu JM, Kim S, Read EJ et al. Engraftment of hematopoietic progenitor cells transduced with the Fanconi Anemia Group C gene (FANCC). Hum Gene Ther 1999; 10(14):2337-2346.
87. Galimi F, Noll M, Kanazawa Y et al. Gene therapy of fanconi anemia by lentiviral vectors. Blood 2002; 100(11):1694.
88. Check E. Second cancer case halts gene-therapy trials. Nature 2003; 421(6921):305.
89. Rabbitts TH, Axelson H, Forster A et al. Chromosomal translocations and leukaemia: A role for LMO2 in T cell acute leukaemia, in transcription and in erythropoiesis. Leukemia 1997; 11(Suppl 3):271-272.
90. Check E. Cancer fears cast doubts on future of gene therapy. Nature 2003; 421(6924):678.
91. Youssoufian H, Kruyt FA, Li X. Protein replacement by receptor-mediated endocytosis corrects the sensitivity of Fanconi anemia group C cells to mitomycin C. Blood 1999; 93(1):363-369.
92. Holmes RK, Harutyunyan K, Shah M et al. Correction of cross-linker sensitivity of Fanconi anemia group F cells by CD33-mediated protein transfer. Blood 2001; 98(13):3817-3822.

CHAPTER 11

Mutational Analyses of Fanconi Anemia Genes in Japanese Patients

Akira Tachibana*

Introduction

Fanconi anemia (FA) is an autosomal recessive disorder characterized by a progressive pancytopenia associated with congenital anomalies and high predisposition to malignancies.[1] Certain FA cell lines are hypersensitive to DNA cross-linking agents such as mitomycin C (MMC) and diepoxybutane (DEB)[2] and has been hypothesized to represent a condition of DNA repair deficiency.[3,4] FA is genetically and clinically heterogeneous. However, the inherited chromosomal instability amplified by DNA cross-linking agents has been a hallmark of this disease. At least 12 complementation groups (FA-A, -B, -C, -D1, -D2, -E, -F, -G, -I, -J, -L, and -M) have been identified by somatic cell hybridization and linkage studied.[5-7] The relative prevalence of each subtype widely varies among ethnic groups; FA-A is predominant in North America and Italy,[8,9] whereas FA-C is most common in Holland, and FA-A and FA-E are equally common in Germany.[10] The genes responsible for these have been identified, that is *FANCA, FANCC, FANCD1/BRCA2, FANCD2, FANCE, FANCF, FANCG, FANCI, FANCJ, FANCL* and *FANCM*.[11-17]

Although relatively large number of patients has been reported in Japan, the genetic basis of FA had remained to be accounted for until recently. The identification of the responsible genes enabled us to assign the FA patients to complementation groups by direct mutation analysis. Since the genetic basis of FA patients in Asian countries is little known, elucidation of the genetic characteristics of Japanese FA contributes the identification of ethnic difference among FA. Furthermore, knowledge of mutation spectra of FA may contribute significantly to the diagnosis and the understanding of pathogenesis of FA. Here, we report mutations in the FA genes among unclassified Japanese FA patients. The preliminary observations have been published elsewhere.[18,19]

Patients, Cell Culture and Mutation Analysis

The patients studied belong to a series that were clinically suspected to be suffering from FA. Peripheral blood samples and skin biopsies from patients have been sent to our laboratory for cytogenetic and genetic diagnosis after consent taken from parents via their clinical doctors. A total of 40 families (45 patients) were confirmed to be suffering from FA by chromosome sensitivity to MMC. For mutation analysis, fibroblast cultures were initiated from skin biopsies and were used for isolation of both genomic DNA and messenger RNA (mRNA) at their early passages. To identify mutations, we employed reverse transcriptase polymerase chain

---

*Akira Tachibana—Radiation Biology Center, Kyoto University, Kyoto 606-8501, Japan.
Email: atachiba@house.rbc.kyoto-u.ac.jp

Molecular Mechanisms of Fanconi Anemia, edited by Shamim I. Ahmad and Sandra H. Kirk.
©2006 Eurekah.com and Springer Science+Business Media.

Table 1. Pathogenic mutations in the FANCA gene

Patient	Mutant Allele 1[a]	Mutant Allele 2[a]
FA18P	1811delT (20)	2546delC (27)
FA20P	1A>G (1)	1A>G (1)
FA23P	3766-3828del (38)	3766-3828del (38)
FA25P	IVS27-1G>A (28)	?
FA28P	1237C>T (14)	4218A>T (42)
FA33P	1A>T (1)	IVS27-2A>T (28)
FA38P	2546delC (27)	2546delC (27)
FA46P	3766-3828del (38)	3766-3828del (38)
AP07P	2152-2778del (24-28)	2546delC (27)
AP22P	2546delC (27)	IVS41-2A>G (42)
AP23P	IVS27-2A>T (28)	?
AP31P	IVS26+134A>G (26)	IVS27-2A>T (28)
AP35P	2546delC (27)	IVS41-2A>G (42)
AP36P	2546delC (27)	IVS27-1G>A (28)
AP38P	2546delC (27)	2546delC (27)
AP48P	1303C>T (14)	1303C>T (14)
AP49P	2546delC (27)	?
AP63P	2546delC (27)	3245T>C (33)
AP68P	1303C>T (14)	2546delC (27)
AP78P	1360-2014del (15-22)[b]	1360-2014del (15-22)[b]

[a] Exons in which the mutations locate are indicated in parentheses. [b] Homozygous in cDNA, but heterozygous in genomic DNA

reaction (RT-PCR) of mRNA and genomic DNA PCR, followed by direct sequencing as described previously.[18]

Sequence Variations in the *FANCA* Gene

Mutations in the *FANCA* gene were screened in 40 unclassified Japanese FA families (45 FA patients and 24 nonFA family members) by sequencing the cDNA including 5' and 3' untranslated regions in both directions, with confirmation by PCR and sequencing of genomic DNA. Altogether 30 sequence alterations were detected; they include 21 base substitutions, two frameshift mutations, three genomic large deletions, and four splicing defects. As the *FANCA* gene has been reported to be highly polymorphic,[20,21] we tested whether a base substitution found in FA patients existed in nonFA controls by RFLP analysis or by direct sequencing. From these analyses, 15 base substitutions were classified as polymorphic variants. They provided suitable markers for haplotype analysis of the patients. Six base substitutions, except for those at the polymorphic sites, all of which are missense mutations, are likely to be pathogenic. Other mutations could be pathogenic because they would cause disruptions of the function of the encoded protein by truncation or deletion in the polypeptide. In all, 15 pathogenic mutations were identified in 20 of 40 FA families (50%). They are listed in Table 1, and the schematic diagram of the distribution is presented in Figure 1. Their primary mutational characteristics and possible functional consequences are described in the following.

Base Substitutions

Two base substitutions found in patients FA20P and FA33P were at the first letter of the start codon (1A>G, 1A>T). These two mutations may totally disrupt the gene function because normal translation may not start at this codon. A new ATG codon appears 172 bp

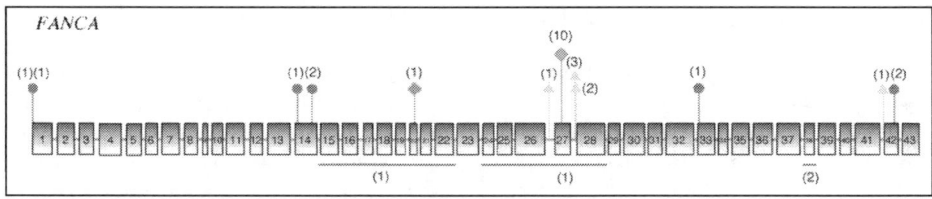

Figure 1. The distribution of pathogenic mutations in the *FANCA* gene. The *FANCA* exons are drawn to scale relative to each other; introns are not shown true to scale. Mutations are shown as follows; base substitution: circle, frameshift: diamond, splicing mutation: triangle, deletion: horizontal bar beneath the gene. Number of patients who harbor the mutation is indicated in brackets.

downstream and runs for only seven codons to terminate after creating a totally dissimilar peptide. Thus, these are likely to be pathogenic mutations. Patient FA20P was homozygous for 1A>G, but heterozygous for a polymorphic site at 1235 (1235C/T), suggesting that the patient received this mutation from both parents.

A missense mutation 1303C>T (R435C) was apparently homozygous in patient AP48P and heterozygous in patient AP68P. The same mutation was reported by Levran et al[20] in a Brazilian patient as a pathogenic mutation. As patient AP48P was homozygous at all the polymorphic sites in the *FANCA* locus, it is not conclusive whether this patient retained the mutation 1303C>T homozygously or hemizygously with a large deletion in the other allele.

Other base substitutions found were 1237C>T (R413C), 3245T>C (L1082P), and 4218A>T (L1406F). Two patients, FA28P and AP63P, were compound heterozygous for these mutations. Both 1237C>T and 1303C>T mutations result in an amino acid change from arginine to cysteine. This amino acid change may be causing an alteration in the protein structure, because arginine is the most basic amino acid, whereas cysteine is rather nonpolar hydrophobic amino acid. The mutation 3245T>C results in the change from leucine to proline. A proline residue may disrupt the normal organization of the backbone of a polypeptide because its side chain is bonded to the nitrogen atom of the amino group. Therefore, this amino acid change will cause a large alteration in the protein structure, which can affect the activity of the gene product. The mutation 4218A>T results in a change from leucine to phenylalanine. Although both amino acids are hydrophobic, this alteration might cause some changes in protein structure or activity, since phenylalanine has an aromatic side chain.

Frameshifts

The 2546delC is a deletion of C moiety within the homonucleotide tract of T in exon 27. This would result in a frameshift and premature termination at 40 codons downstream that predicts a truncated protein of 887 amino acids. This mutation was most common among the pathogenic mutations, being found in 10 of 40 FA patients. Two patients, FA38P and AP38P, appeared homozygous for this mutation, suggesting that they retained this mutation homozygously. However, it is also possible that these patients harbor this mutation on one allele together with a deletion on the other allele. For example, analysis of the family members of AP38P revealed that the father (AP38F) was heterozygous for this mutation, but the mother (AP38M) showed only wild-type sequence at this site. We have not identified the mutation in AP38M, but it could be a large deletion. Another frameshift mutation is 1811delT in exon 20 found in FA18P. This would results in a premature termination producing a truncated protein of 606 amino acids.

RNA Splicing Mutations

Four mutations affecting RNA splicing were identified. Splicing potential was estimated by calculating the splice site score ("*s*") following the formulas described by Shapiro and Senapathy,[22] using the tabulated nucleotide frequencies.[23] IVS26+134A>G was an A>G transition at 134 bp downstream from exon 26, resulting in an mRNA with an insertion of 129 bp between exon 26 and exon 27 (2504ins129). This mutation modulates the potential of a pseudo-splice donor site at 130 bp downstream from exon 26 from $s = 65.3$ to $s = 79.8$, which is similar to that of the intrinsic splice donor site ($s = 79.6$), resulting in the insertion of 129 bp to exon 26 in cDNA. The inserted sequence creates a new stop codon 2 bp downstream from the tail of exon 26, resulting in a truncated protein of 835 amino acids. Two mutations, IVS27-2A>T and IVS27-1G>A, were identified at the splice acceptor site of exon 28. Analysis of cDNA sequence showed that both alterations caused a 6-bp deletion in cDNA (2602-2607del), resulted in an in-frame deletion of two amino acids (Phe, Gln), i.e., 868-869delFQ. Both mutations lead to the reduction of the splice site score of the authentic site from $s = 88.5$ to $s = 72.6$. The splice score of a cryptic splice acceptor site in exon 28 that resides 6 bp downstream from the 5' end of the exon is 88.5 in normal sequence. The splice site score of this cryptic splice site has risen to 92.7 by IVS27-2A>T, although IVS27-1G>A does not affect the score. Therefore, both mutations inactivate the intrinsic splice acceptor site, resulting in the aberrant splicing to the cryptic splice site in exon 28. Another splice-site mutation was found at the splice acceptor site in intron 41 (IVS41-2A>G) that caused a reduction in splice site score from $s = 90.1$ to $s = 74.2$, resulting in an in-frame skipping of exon 42 (4168-4260del). This would produce a truncated protein with 1,424 amino acids.

Deletions

A homozygous loss of exon 38 (3766-3828del) was observed in the cDNA of two patients, FA23P and FA46P, causing an in-frame deletion of 21 amino acids. In these patients, PCR amplification of exon 38 for genomic DNA did not show any amplified product, indicating a homozygous genomic deletion involving exon 38. Amplification of the genetic region from exon 37 to exon 39 of both patients generated an approximately 1.8-kb fragment. Sequence analysis showed that both patients had the identical deletion. The 5' breakpoint of the deletion locates at a tail of a homonucleotide tract of A between *SpeI* and *HindIII* sites in intron 37 and the 3' breakpoint locates at 49 bp from the 5' end of exon 38, sharing an A at the junction. This deletion removes the splice acceptor site in intron 37, resulting in the loss of exon 38 in the *FANCA* cDNA. Since both patients were homozygous at polymorphic sites, it is not conclusive whether these patients harbored the homozygous deletion or hemizygous with a much larger deletion in the other allele.

Sequence analysis of cDNA from patient AP07P revealed an altered cDNA that lost a sequence from exon 24 to exon 28 was detected. This alteration (2152-2778del) is an in-frame deletion that removes 209 amino acids from the FANCA protein. From the results of extensive sequence analysis, we concluded that one *FANCA* allele in this patient contains a large genomic deletion involving a region from exon 24 to exon 28. The prediction that 2152-2778del resulted from a genomic deletion and not from a splice-site mutation is substantiated by the results that no sequence alteration was found in the genomic PCR fragments of exons 24 and 28, including their flanking regions.

RT-PCR of the *FANCA* cDNA of patient AP78P revealed a short PCR product in homozygous state. This small cDNA lost a sequence from exon 15 to exon 22 (1360-2014del). This alteration is an in-frame deletion that removed 218 amino acids from the FANCA protein. RT-PCR analysis showed that the father of this patient (AP78F) contained both the small-size and the normal-size cDNA, indicating that the allele that generated this short cDNA was paternal origin. RT-PCR analysis of the mother of this patient (AP78M) showed only the cDNA of normal size. The patient was heterozygous at several polymorphic sites indicating that the patient retained both the paternal and the maternal allele of the *FANCA* locus. However, the patient was homozygous at a polymorphic site (1927C/G) in exon 22, which indicated that the patient retained the maternal allele only in the region. The most probable explanation of these results is that the patient retained a paternal allele that had a deletion from exon 15 to exon 22 and a maternal allele that contained the full length of the gene but was not

Table 2. Nonpathogenic polymorphic sites in the FANCA gene

Sequence Alteration	Exon		Amino Acid Change
796A/G	9	T/A266	Thr/Ala
1049G/A	12	R/Q350	Arg/Gln
1143G/T	13	T/T381	Thr: silent
1235G/T	14	A/V412	Ala/Val
1501A/G	16	S/G501	Ser/Gly
1927C/G	22	P/A643	Pro/Ala
2265A/T	25	G/G755	Gly: silent
2426G/A	26	G/D809	Gly/Asp
2901C/T	30	S/S967	Ser: silent
3114C/T	32	L/L1038	Leu: silent
3114C/G	32	L/L1038	Leu: silent
3654A/G	37	P/P1218	Pro: silent
3807G/C	38	L/L1269	Leu: silent
3982A/G	40	T/A1328	Thr/Ala
4000G/A	40	A/T1334	Ala/Thr

expressed. Since no sequence alteration was identified in the promoter region, the expression of the maternal allele might be reduced by methylation or some other epigenetic mechanism.

Altogether, 15 mutations were assumed to be pathogenic mutations, which were found in 20 of 40 patients (50%). The most common mutation was 2546delC found in 10 patients. This is a remarkable characteristic in Japanese FA-A patients, and is likely to be a founder mutation of Japanese population. In addition to the mutations described above, there could be large deletions that would result in hemizygosity, which could not be identified by the method we employed. The examination of AP78P and the family suggested that the reduction of the gene expression, e.g., by methylation, might also play a role in FA-A pathogenesis.

Nonpathogenic Polymorphic Variants

The *FANCA* gene has been reported to be highly polymorphic.[8,20] In all, 15 polymorphic changes were identified in Japanese patients (Table 2). Seven of them were silent alterations that did not replace amino acids. Two polymorphisms, 3114C/T and 3114C/G were different changes at the same site found in different individuals. Eight base substitutions result in amino acid changes. These base changes were surveyed in nonFA controls either by RFLP analysis where an appropriate restriction site was available, or by direct sequencing of PCR products. 796A/G, 1235C/T, 1501A/G and 2426G/A were those previously assigned to nonpathogenic sequence polymorphism in nonJapanese populations (Fanconi Anemia Mutation Database http://www.rockefeller.edu/fanconi/mutate). 796A/G and 2426G/A may be common variants among the Japanese population because they appeared biallelic in all patients, FA family members and nonFA controls who were analyzed. Since a base substitution variant 3982A/G creates a new restriction site of *Cac8I*, RFLP analysis was performed in 20 nonFA controls. The allele frequency of this variant was 0.075 per normal chromosome, which was not different from that in the FA patients. Therefore, this variant is highly likely to be a benign polymorphism. A base substitution variant 1927C/G is also likely to be a polymorphism because RFLP analysis using restriction enzyme *Mwo*I identified this variant at an allele frequency of 0.075 in the control population, which was similar to 0.10 in the FA patients. It was noted that the cDNA always a significant fraction lacked of exon 30 in all cell lines studied, including those from unaffected family members and normal controls. The skipping of exon 30 may be a leaky alteration associated with an alternative splicing and may not be related to the disease.

Table 3. Pathogenic mutations in the FANCG gene

Patient	Mutant Allele 1[a]	Mutant Allele 2[a]
FA5P	IVS3+1G>C (3)	1066C>T (8)
FA9P	IVS3+1G>C (3)	IVS3+1G>C (3)
FA14P	1066C>T (8)	1066C>T (8)
FA17P	IVS3+1G>C (3)	IVS3+1G>C (3)
FA21P	IVS3+1G>C (3)	IVS3+1G>C (3)
FA24P	IVS13-2A>G (14)	IVS13-2A>G (14)
FA29P	IVS13-2A>G (14)	IVS13-2A>G (14)
FA31P	IVS3+1G>C (3)	IVS3+1G>C (3)
FA32P	IVS3+1G>C (3)	IVS3+1G>C (3)
AP02P	IVS3+1G>C (3)	1066C>T (8)
AP66P	IVS3+1G>C (3)	IVS3+1G>C (3)
AP74P	IVS3+1G>C (3)	1066C>T (8)

[a] Exons in which the mutations locate are indicated in parentheses.

Sequence Variations in the *FANCG* Gene

Twenty patients were thus assigned to FA-A by mutation analysis of the *FANCA* gene. Then, we analyzed the *FANCG* gene in the remaining 20 nonFA-A patients using RT-PCR analysis. Gel electrophoresis analysis of the PCR products revealed amplified products in all patients, and some showed small bands.

Direct sequencing of the RT-PCR products revealed three types of sequence alterations in cDNA in 12 of the 20 patients (Table 3). Among these, RT-PCR analysis showed that six patients had two cDNA species; both were shorter than normal band with no trace of normal band. Direct sequencing of cDNA showed that these two short bands corresponded to the skipping of exon 3 (176-307del) and the skipping of exons 3 and 4 (176-510del), respectively. Cloning and sequencing of RT-PCR products confirmed these two alterations. The ratio of the 176-307del clones to the 176-510del clones was 9 to 11, being consistent with the 1:1 ratio. Sequencing of the region of genomic DNA from exon 1 to exon 7 detected one homozygous base substitution at the splice donor site of intron 3 (IVS3+1G>C). Therefore, this alteration resulted in two alternative splicing events. The sequence change causes the reduction of the splice site score from $s = 93.5$ to $s = 75.3$. The deletion 176-307del in cDNA removes entire exon 3 of 132 bp, resulting in an in-frame deletion of 44 amino acids. The deletion 176-510del removes both exon 3 and exon 4, deleting 335 bp that yields an out-of-frame mRNA with a termination codon TAA at new codon 63. This mutation was detected in 9 patients, apparently homozygous in 6 patients and heterozygous in 3 patients. Among the homozygous patients, family analyses were available for 2 patients (FA31P and AP66P). RT-PCR and genomic PCR followed by sequencing analysis revealed that both parents of both families were heterozygous for IVS3+1G>C. Thus, the patient FA31P and AP66P was homozygous for IVS3+1G>C rather than hemizygous for the mutation. As we have no information on family members of the other 4 apparently homozygous patients, it is unclear whether they were homozygous or hemizygous. Both RT-PCR gel electrophoresis patterns and sequencing profiles showed no trace amount of alternatively spliced products in normal control individuals. Furthermore, since IVS3+1G>C creates a new restriction site of *DdeI*, RFLP analysis was performed in 20 nonFA controls. No alteration was identified in control individuals.

Sequence analysis of RT-PCR products revealed a homozygous 20-bp deletion (1761-1780del) in 2 patients (FA24P and FA29P), which corresponded to the deletion of the 5' end of exon 14. This alteration causes a stop codon at 587, resulting in a truncated protein.

Genomic DNA analysis showed a homozygous mutation at the splice acceptor site in intron 13 (IVS13-2A>G). This mutation is similar to the IVS13-1G>C mutation reported previously[14] in a consanguineous Lebanese family. Both IVS13-2A>G and IVS13-1G>C mutations reduced the splice site score from $s = 91.4$ to $s = 75.5$, whereas the score of the cryptic splice site at 1781 remained unchanged ($s = 75.6$). Both mutations will cause the alteration of splicing at the splice acceptor site of exon 14, which results in the same truncated protein.

Another sequence alteration identified in cDNA was 1059-1076del, removing 18 nucleotides from the 3' end of exon 8. This alteration resulted in a deletion of 6 amino acids in the *FANCG* gene product. Sequence analysis of genomic DNA showed a heterozygous C>T substitution at position +142 in exon 8 (1066C>T). The corresponding amino acid alteration was a substitution of a termination codon (X) for glutamine (Q) at codon 356 (Q356X) in the characterized coding sequence for *FANCG*. This base substitution located at 11 bp upstream from the end of exon 8, and was not present in the cDNA, as the sequence containing this mutation was spliced out from the mRNA. The mutation was identified in 4 patients, apparently homozygous in one patient (FA14P) and heterozygous in 3 patients. Family analysis showed that the mother of the patient (AP02M) had 176-307del and 176-510del in cDNA and was heterozygous for IVS3+1G>C, while the father (AP02F) had 1059-1076del in cDNA and was heterozygous for 1066C>T in genomic DNA. No sequence alteration was found in the genomic *FANCG* exon 8 of 20 unrelated control individuals, suggesting the pathogenic nature of this base substitution.

We have identified three polymorphic changes in the *FANCG* gene. 890C/T in exon 7, which had been reported as a polymorphic site previously,[24] was found in an FA-A patient (AP35P) and a nonFA control. 1845T/C, which has no effect on amino acid sequence, was detected heterozygously in an FA-A patient (FA25P) and an unclassified FA patient (FA12P). IVS1+77A/C is a polymorphism in intron 1, which has no effect on the coding sequence. This polymorphism was detected in 2 FA-G patients (AP02P and AP66P) and an FA-A patient (AP68P). Although we have not analyzed completely, this polymorphism might be very common in Japanese population.

In all, *FANCG* mutations were found in 12 out of a total of 40 Japanese patients (30%). The splicing mutation IVS3+1G>C is the most common mutation in Japanese FA-G patients. Therefore, this mutation might be a founder mutation of Japanese population. Nine patients were apparently homozygous for these mutations; two of them were confirmed to be homozygous by the analysis of family members. However, as the zygosity for the other patients was not conclusive, they might be either homozygous for the mutations or hemizygous with the mutation and a deletion on another allele. Although the number of patients is considerably large, only three pathogenic mutations were identified in our panel of Japanese patients. Recently, Yagasaki et al[25] reported the *FANCG* mutations in 10 families of 45 Japanese patients (22%). They also reported that IVS3+1G>C was the most common mutation. In addition, mutations 91C>T and 194delC were identified. Altogether, only 5 *FANCG* mutations have been identified in Japanese patients, as shown in Figure 2. This is in marked contrast to the result on 58 FA patients mainly from North America, which detected 27 mutations distributing over the entire *FANCG* gene.[26]

The 1066C>T mutation is noteworthy because of the alteration found in mRNA. It is anticipated that this base substitution will cause a substitution of a termination codon for glutamine (Q) at codon 356 (Q356X). However, RT-PCR analysis of the mRNA from the 2 patients showed an 18-bp deletion at the end of exon 8 (1059-1076del), resulting in an in-frame deletion of 6 codons in the *FANCG* gene product. Since this mutation is located at 11 bp upstream from the end of exon 8 in genomic DNA, it is removed from the patient's mRNA, and does not result in a truncation of the gene product. Therefore, it was assumed that this mutation affected the splicing by altering the splice site score at a cryptic splicing donor site. However, the splice site scores at both the cryptic donor site at position 1058 and the authentic donor site were not altered by the mutation. These results suggest that the mutation 1066C>T

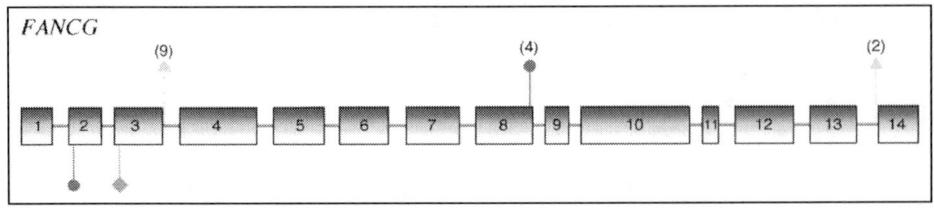

Figure 2. The distribution of pathogenic mutations in the *FANCG* gene. The *FANCG* exons are drawn to scale relative to each other; introns are not shown true to scale. Mutations are shown as follows; base substitution: circle, frameshift: diamond, splicing mutation: triangle. Mutations identified in our laboratory are indicated above the gene with the number of patients who harbor the mutation in brackets. Two new mutations reported by Yagasaki et al[24] are shown beneath the gene.

that would cause a premature termination codon (PTC) affects some splicing step(s) without altering the splicing site score.

PTC-bearing mRNAs are a problem for cells, as they encode truncated proteins, some of which possess dominant-negative or deleterious gain-of-function activity. It is estimated that 30% of inherited genetic disorders in humans result from PTC mutations.[27] To prevent the production of such deleterious truncated proteins from nonsense codon containing mRNA, two cellular responses have been defined. One is nonsense-mediated mRNA decay (NMD), a pathway that degrades mRNAs harboring nonsense codons.[28] The second is nonsense-associated altered splicing (NAS), a response that increases the levels of alternatively spliced transcripts that have skipped the termination codons.[29,30] It has been assumed that NMD and NAS are regulated by the same mechanism since both of them require both a nonsense codon and a translation-like process. However, it was recently shown that NMD and NAS are distinct mechanisms.[31,32] The mutation 1066C>T would cause the alteration in RNA splicing through NMD or NAS. By cloning and sequencing the *FANCG* cDNA of patient FA14P who is homozygous for 1066C>T, we detected cDNA with 18-bp deletion only and no full-length cDNA. Although this result prefers NAS, we reserve conclusion on the mechanism for the formation of alternative splicing.

The same cryptic splice donor site in exon 8 was used by another splicing mutation as described previously.[26] The IVS8-2A>G mutation, the most common mutation in Portuguese Brazilian,[24,26] is predicted to result in the loss of exon 9 because of the inactivation of the intron 8 acceptor site. Analysis of cDNA by RT-PCR and sequencing revealed cDNAs using two cryptic splice donor sites in exon 8. One of them was the cryptic site at position 1058. Therefore, two mutations, 1066C>T and IVS8-2A>G, result in the usage of the same cryptic site.

Altered splicing caused by a premature termination codon usually results in skipping of one or more exons in most cases. For instance, Gibson et al reported that a nonsense mutation in exon 6 of the *FANCC* gene (808C>T) caused skipping of exon 6 in about half of the RT-PCR products of the *FANCC* gene.[33] The mutation of 1066C>T in the *FANCG* gene is unique, as the nonsense mutation resulted in the skipping of part of the exon, not the entire exon, utilizing the cryptic splice donor site near the nonsense codon. Therefore, the 1066C>T mutation might be intriguing for the study of RNA splicing and the nonsense surveillance mechanism.

Recommendations for a nomenclature system for human gene mutations[34] describe to indicate the nucleotide position in cDNA for a mutation found in exon. However, this will be misleading in some cases, such as the *FANCG* mutation 1066C>T and the *FANCC* mutation 808C>T. The representation such as "1066C>T" or "808C>T" indicates a termination codon, not a deletion, in mRNA, although the real outcome is a skipping of a part of or an entire exon in mRNA. According to the updated nomenclature recommendation,[35] the 1066C>T mutation can be described as "g. 1066C>T" and "c. 1059-1076del". Although the updated

Mutations of the *FANCC* Gene

We next analyzed mutation of the *FANCC* gene in the remaining 8 nonA/nonG patients, using RT-PCR and direct sequencing of the *FANCC* cDNA. No sequence alteration was detected in the *FANCC* gene in all patients (data not shown). This result contrasts to the recent observations,[36] which reported mutations of the *FANCC* gene in 9 of 24 unrelated Japanese FA patients. They identified the IVS4+4A>T mutation homozygous in 8 patients and heterozygous in one patient. Our observations indicate that the proportion of FA-C patients in Japanese population may be very small, if any at all.

Mutations of Other FA Genes

We also analyzed mutations in the nonA/nonG/nonC patients for other FA genes, i.e., *FANCD2*, *FANCE* and *FANCF* genes.[7,15,16] However, analyses using RT-PCR and sequencing revealed no pathologically meaningful mutations in these 8 patients who have been preexcluded for the mutations at the *FANCA*, *FANCG* and *FANCC* genes. Because of the high accuracy in detecting mutations by direct sequencing of entire coding region, FA-D2, -E and -F are unlikely for these patients as well.

Recently, the responsible gene for FA-D1 was identified as the *BRCA2* gene.[17] We confirmed that one of our unclassified FA patient (AP37P) was compound heterozygous for mutations of the *BRCA2/FANCD1* gene. Search for mutations in other unclassified Japanese patients is undergoing.

Characteristics and Genetic Basis of Japanese FA Patients

We have screened 40 unrelated Japanese FA families for mutations in 7 FA genes by direct sequencing of cDNA with confirmation on genomic DNA. Twenty of them (50%) retained mutations in the *FANCA* gene, 12 (30%) retained mutations in the *FANCG* gene, and one (2.5%) in the *BRCA2/FANCD1* gene. Although there is a report on the high prevalence of *FANCC* mutation in Japanese patients,[36] our analysis failed to detect any mutations in the *FANCC* gene, including the reported mutation of IVS4+4A>T. Futaki et al[36] studied 24 unrelated patients by polymerase chain reaction and single strand conformation polymorphism (PCR-SSCP) strategy and found the IVS4+4A>T mutation, which had been previously reported in Ashkenazi-Jewish patients,[37] in 9 patients (38 %). The reason of the discrepancy is unknown. One possible explanation for this discrepancy might be a sampling bias. In general, however, the proportion of the FA-C patients in Japanese FA might be considerably small, if any at all. Recently, Yagasaki et al[25] studied *FANCG* mutations in 45 unrelated Japanese families and found mutations in 10 families (22 %), where IVS3+1G>C splice mutations predominated. Our observations are consistent with their observations.

The International Fanconi Anemia Registry collects FA patients; most of them are from North America, and some from Brazil, India, and Turkey. Complementation groups FA-A (65%), FA-C (15%), and FA-G (10%) account for the majority of FA patients in the Registry.[20,38-41] Our results showed that FA-A is the most prevailing among Japanese patients as the Western countries, but the difference is rather higher prevalence of FA-G and possible paucity of FA-C as compared with those in Western countries.

In spite of the comprehensive survey by direct sequencing strategy for mutations of possible FA-related genes, at least 7 of 40 patients (17.5%) still remain unclassified. They are not distinct from other patients in their clinical manifestation and chromosomal sensitivity to MMC. They could be due to mutations of other genes, e.g., *FANCB*, or perturbed expression of known gene(s) by methylation modification or other epigenetic mechanisms. The repair pathway for DNA interstrand crosslinks (ICL) is complex and not well understood in higher eukaryotes. Studies in *Escherichia coli* and yeast indicate that both nucleotide excision repair (NER) and homologous recombination are required for ICL removal.[42] A combined participation of NER and recombination was also suggested for mammalian cells.[42] In particular, a central role was suggested for the NER excinuclease heterodimer XPF-ERCC1.[43-45] Indeed, in addition to the cooperative functioning among the FA gene products,[46-48] other genes are also suggested to play a part in ICL repair, such as *BRCA1*[49] and RAD50/MRE11/NBS1.[50,51] Moreover, FANCA protein was recently reported to colocalize with nonerythroid α spectrin and XPF protein to the same nuclear foci upon ICL damage.[52] Since FA proteins form a very complex interaction with other proteins, any change in the interaction might affect the ICL repair, which in turn may cause an FA phenotype.

Although the proportion of FA-A in Japanese FA patients is relatively high, genetic analysis of the *FANCA* gene is rather laborious. The gene is considerably large; it is about 4.5 kb in cDNA, and consists of 43 exons. Moreover, the mutations, together with polymorphic variants, distribute throughout the entire gene. FA-G is the second largest group in Japanese patients, and there seems very limited diversity in mutation spectrum of the *FANCG* gene. Particularly, IVS3+1G>C is the most common mutation in FA-G. Therefore, for the genetic diagnosis of Japanese FA patients, mutation analysis of the *FANCG* gene, above all the IVS3+1G>C mutation, could be a primary choice. When no mutation was identified in the *FANCG* gene, survey of the *FANCA* mutation may be suggested. Since the 2546delC is the most common *FANCA* mutation in Japanese patients, analysis of this mutation might be useful, but as the mutations distribute throughout the *FANCA* gene, survey of the entire gene is necessary.

Acknowledgments

I thank Dr. Masao S. Sasaki, Professor Emeritus, Kyoto University, for his critical reading of the manuscript and valuable comments. Thanks are also due to Dr. Toshiko Yamada and Mrs. Noriko Hirayama for their excellent technical assistance. This work was supported in part by Grants in Aid from the Ministry of Education, Culture, Sports, Science and Technology of Japan and the Ministry of Health, Labour and Welfare of Japan.

References

1. Butturini A, Gale RP, Verlander PC et al. Hematologic abnormalities in fanconi anemia: An international fanconi anemia registry study. Blood 1994; 84:1650-1655.
2. Sasaki MS, Tonomura A. A high susceptibility of Fanconi's anemia to chromosome breakage by DNA cross-linking agents. Cancer Res 1973; 33:1829-1836.
3. Sasaki MS. Is Fanconi's anaemia defective in a process essential to the repair of DNA cross links? Nature 1975; 257:501-503.
4. Sasaki MS. Fanconi's anemia: A condition possibly associated with a defective DNA repair. In: Hanawalt PC, Friedberg EC, Fox CF, eds. DNA repair mechanisms. New York: Academic Press, 1978:675-684.
5. Joenje H, Oostra AB, Wijker M et al. Evidence for at least eight Fanconi anemia genes. Am J Hum Genet 1997; 61:940-944.
6. Joenje H, Levitus M, Waisfisz Q et al. Complementation analysis in Fanconi anemia: Assignment of the reference FA-H patient to group A. Am J Hum Genet 2000; 67:759-762.
7. Timmers C, Taniguchi T, Hejna J et al. Positional cloning of a novel Fanconi anemia gene, FANCD2. Mol Cell 2001; 7:241-248.
8. Savoia A, Zatterale A, Del Principe D et al. Fanconi anaemia in Italy: High prevalence of complementation group A in two geographic clusters. Hum Genet 1996; 97:599.
9. Jakobs PM, Fiddler-Odell E, Reifsteck C et al. Complementation group assignments in Fanconi anemia fibroblast cell lines from North America. Somat Cell Mol Genet 1997; 23:1-7.
10. Joenje H. Fanconi anaemia complementation groups in Germany and the Netherlands. Hum Genet 1996; 97:280-282.
11. Strathdee CA, Gavish H, Shannon WR et al. Cloning of cDNAs for Fanconi's anaemia by functional complementation. Nature 1992; 356:763-767.
12. The fanconi anemia/breast cancer consortium positional cloning of the fanconi anaemia group A gene. Nat Genet 1996; 14:324.
13. Lo Ten Foe JR, Rooimans MA, Bosnoyan-Collins L et al. Expression cloning of a cDNA for the major Fanconi anaemia gene, FAA. Nat Genet 1996; 14:320-323.

14. de Winter JP, Waisfisz Q, Rooimans MA et al. The Fanconi anaemia group G gene FANCG is identical with XRCC9. Nat Genet 1998; 20:281-283.
15. de Winter JP, Leveille F, van Berkel CG et al. Isolation of a cDNA representing the Fanconi anemia complementation group E gene. Am J Hum Genet 2000; 67:1306-1308.
16. de Winter JP, Rooimans MA, van Der Weel L et al. The Fanconi anaemia gene FANCF encodes a novel protein with homology to ROM. Nat Genet 2000; 24:15-16.
17. Howlett NG, Taniguchi T, Olson S et al. Biallelic inactivation of BRCA2 in Fanconi anemia. Science 2002; 297:606-609.
18. Tachibana A, Kato T, Ejima Y et al. The FANCA gene in Japanese Fanconi anemia: Reports of eight novel mutations and analysis of sequence variability. Hum Mutat 1999; 13:237-244.
19. Yamada T, Tachibana A, Shimizu T et al. Novel mutations of the FANCG gene causing alternative splicing in Japanese Fanconi anemia. J Hum Genet 2000; 45:159-166.
20. Levran O, Erlich T, Magdalena N et al. Sequence variation in the Fanconi anemia gene FAA. Proc Natl Acad Sci USA 1997; 94:13051-13056.
21. Savino M, Ianzano L, Strippoli P et al. Mutations of the Fanconi anemia group A gene (FAA) in Italian patients. Am J Hum Genet 1997; 61:1246-1253.
22. Shapiro MB, Senapathy P. RNA splice junctions of different classes of eukaryotes: Sequence statistics and functional implications in gene expression. Nucleic Acids Res 1987; 15:7155-7174.
23. Senapathy P, Shapiro MB, Harris NL. Splice junctions, branchpoint sites, and exons: Sequence statistics, identification, and applications to genome project. Methods in Enzymology. New York: Academic Press, 1990:252.
24. Demuth I, Wlodarski M, Tipping AJ et al. Spectrum of mutations in the Fanconi anaemia group G gene, FANCG/XRCC9. Eur J Hum Genet 2000; 8:861-868.
25. Yagasaki H, Oda T, Adachi D et al. Two common founder mutations of the fanconi anemia group G gene FANCG/XRCC9 in the Japanese population. Hum Mutat 2003; 21:555.
26. Auerbach AD, Greenbaum J, Pujara K et al. Spectrum of sequence variation in the FANCG gene: An International Fanconi anemia Registry (IFAR) study. Hum Mutat 2003; 21:158-168.
27. Frischmeyer PA, Dietz HC. Nonsense-mediated mRNA decay in health and disease. Hum Mol Genet 1999; 8:1893-1900.
28. Maquat LE. When cells stop making sense: Effects of nonsense codons on RNA metabolism in vertebrate cells. RNA 1995; 1:453-465.
29. Valentine CR. The association of nonsense codons with exon skipping. Mutat Res 1998; 411:87-117.
30. Maquat LE. NASty effects on fibrillin premRNA splicing: Another case of ESE does it, but proposals for translation-dependent splice site choice live on. Genes Dev 2002; 16:1743-1753.
31. Mendell JT, Ap Rhys CM, Dietz HC. Separable roles for rent1/hUpf1 in altered splicing and decay of nonsense transcripts. Science 2002; 298:419-422.
32. Wang J, Chang YF, Hamilton JI et al. Nonsense-associated altered splicing: A frame-dependent response distinct from nonsense-mediated decay. Mol Cell 2002; 10:951-957.
33. Gibson RA, Hajianpour A, Murer-Orlando M et al. A nonsense mutation and exon skipping in the Fanconi anaemia group C gene. Hum Mol Genet 1993; 2:797-799.
34. Antonarakis SE. And the Nomenclature working group recommendations for a nomenclature system for human gene mutations. Nomenclature Working Group. Hum Mutat 1998; 11:1-3.
35. den Dunnen JT, Antonarakis SE. Nomenclature for the description of human sequence variations. Hum Genet 2001; 109:121-124.
36. Futaki M, Yamashita T, Yagasaki H et al. The IVS4 + 4 A to T mutation of the fanconi anemia gene FANCC is not associated with a severe phenotype in Japanese patients. Blood 2000; 95:1493-1498.
37. Whitney MA, Saito H, Jakobs PM et al. A common mutation in the FACC gene causes Fanconi anaemia in Ashkenazi Jews. Nat Genet 1993; 4:202-205.
38. Verlander PC, Lin JD, Udono MU et al. Mutation analysis of the Fanconi anemia gene FACC. Am J Hum Genet 1994; 54:595-601.
39. Verlander PC, Kaporis A, Liu Q et al. Carrier frequency of the IVS4 + 4 A—>T mutation of the Fanconi anemia gene FAC in the Ashkenazi Jewish population. Blood 1995; 86:4034-4038.
40. Gillio AP, Verlander PC, Batish SD et al. Phenotypic consequences of mutations in the Fanconi anemia FAC gene: An international fanconi anemia registry study. Blood 1997; 90:105-110.
41. Levran O, Doggett NA, Auerbach AD. Identification of Alu-mediated deletions in the Fanconi anemia gene FAA. Hum Mutat 1998; 12:145-152.
42. Dronkert ML, Kanaar R. Repair of DNA interstrand cross-links. Mutat Res 2001; 486:217-247.
43. Hoy CA, Thompson LH, Mooney CL et al. Defective DNA cross-link removal in Chinese hamster cell mutants hypersensitive to bifunctional alkylating agents. Cancer Res 1985; 45:1737-1743.

44. De Silva IU, McHugh PJ, Clingen PH et al. Defining the roles of nucleotide excision repair and recombination in the repair of DNA interstrand cross-links in mammalian cells. Mol Cell Biol 2000; 20:7980-7990.
45. Wang X, Peterson CA, Zheng H et al. Involvement of nucleotide excision repair in a recombination-independent and error-prone pathway of DNA interstrand cross-link repair. Mol Cell Biol 2001; 21:713-720.
46. Grompe M, D'Andrea A. Fanconi anemia and DNA repair. Hum Mol Genet 2001; 10:2253-2259.
47. Joenje H, Patel KJ. The emerging genetic and molecular basis of Fanconi anaemia. Nat Rev Genet 2001; 2:446-457.
48. Bagby Jr GC. Genetic basis of Fanconi anemia. Curr Opin Hematol 2003; 10:68-76.
49. Garcia-Higuera I, Taniguchi T, Ganesan S et al. Interaction of the Fanconi anemia proteins and BRCA1 in a common pathway. Mol Cell 2001; 7:249-262.
50. Nakanishi K, Taniguchi T, Ranganathan V et al. Interaction of FANCD2 and NBS1 in the DNA damage response. Nat Cell Biol 2002; 4:913-920.
51. Pichierri P, Averbeck D, Rosselli F. DNA cross-link-dependent RAD50/MRE11/NBS1 subnuclear assembly requires the Fanconi anemia C protein. Hum Mol Genet 2002; 11:2531-2546.
52. Sridharan D, Brown M, Lambert WC et al. Nonerythroid αII spectrin is required for recruitment of FANCA and XPF to nuclear foci induced by DNA interstrand cross-links. J Cell Sci 2003; 116:823-835.

Index

Symbols

9p13 14, 20, 56
16q24.3 14, 28
176-307del 108, 109
176-307del clones 108
176-510del 108, 109
176-510del clones 108
322delG 8, 16, 18, 39, 40, 45, 46, 48, 49
796A/G 107
808C>T 110
868-869delFQ 106
890C/T 109
890C/T in exon 7 109
1059-1076del 109, 110
1066C>T 108-110
1066C>T mutation 109, 110
1235C/T 105, 107
1360-2014del 104, 106
1501A/G 107
1927C/G 106, 107
(1927C/G) in exon 22 106
2426G/A 107
2546delC 104, 105, 107, 112
3114C/G 107
3114C/T 107

A

α spectrin II 78
A-T 1-3, 5, 9, 10, 16
Acute myeloid leukemia (AML) 3, 4, 7-9, 13, 28, 32, 33, 40, 93
Acute nonlymphocytic leukemia 13
Adeno-associated virus (AAV) 96, 97
Adenosine deaminase 95
Adenoviruses 96
AKT 14
Akt kinase 77, 79
Alpha spectrin 16, 42
Alpha-tocopherol 83
Alu repeat sequences 29
AML/MDS 8
Androgens 4, 92, 94
Anti-FANCA antibody 69
Antioxidant 47, 48, 82-85
Antithymocyte globulin (ATG) 36, 93-96, 104
Aplastic anemia 1, 3-7, 13, 92, 93, 95, 96
Apoptosis 17, 32, 41-49, 75, 76, 79, 82, 97
Arabidopsis 61
Ashkenazi Jewish 10, 16, 29, 40
ASK signaling 18
ASK1 17, 18, 48, 49
αSPIIΣ* 42, 78
Ataxia telangiectasia 1, 10, 62, 63
ATLD 5
ATM 2, 9, 10, 55, 63, 64
ATM kinase 63
ATR checkpoint kinase 19, 87
Autosomal 1, 36, 54, 67, 103
Autoubiquitination 70
Azathioprine 96

B

BARD1 62
BASC complex 63, 64
BLM 2, 21, 22, 55, 64, 70
Bloom syndrome (BS) 1, 2, 6, 70
Bone marrow (BM) 1, 3, 4, 7-9, 13, 15, 17, 20, 29, 30, 32, 37, 41, 43-48, 67, 75, 82, 84, 86, 87, 92-94, 96-98
Bone marrow failure 1, 3, 4, 7, 9, 13, 15, 29, 30, 32, 46, 75, 82, 84, 86, 87, 92, 97
Bone marrow transplant (BMT) 4, 30, 93-95, 98
Brazilian patient 105
BRCA1 2, 14, 16, 19, 21, 47, 58, 61-64, 68, 69, 75, 76, 78, 79, 112
BRCA2 2, 4, 7-10, 13, 14, 16, 18, 19, 21, 22, 55-58, 61-64, 68-70, 74, 79, 87, 103, 111
Breast cancer 9, 62-64, 75
BRG1 15, 16, 75, 76
BTB/POZ 75
Burst forming units-erythrocytes (BFU-E) 45, 93

C

c. 1059-1076del 110
C. elegans 61
CAAT box 37
Café au lait 5, 9
Carcinomas 1, 3, 4, 6, 8, 33, 95
Caspase 41, 45-47, 76
Caspase-3 activation 45-47
Catalase 83-85
CD4 17
CD33 98
CD34+ 37, 41, 42, 44, 45, 93-95, 97
CD34+ *Fancc*-/- 44
CD95 44, 45
Cdc2 16, 42, 43, 75
Cdc2 kinase 42, 43
cDNA 6, 14, 28, 36, 37, 39, 40, 43, 44, 46, 56, 61, 67, 104, 106-112
cDNA library 37
Central nervous system (CNS) 5, 8, 40, 54
Chromatin 2, 15, 16, 18, 21, 22, 42, 75, 78
Chromosome abnormalities 1, 2, 9
Chromosome 7 7
Chromosome 14 7
Cis-platin 43, 82, 83
CK-2 39
Clinical trial 97
Clonogenic assays 97
CNS defects 40
CNS malformations 8
Coding sequence include G139E 40
Colony forming units-granulocyte-macrophage (CFU-GM) 93
Combined immunodeficiency disease 98
Complementation analysis 6, 7, 14, 39, 54, 69
CpG methylation-induced mutation 29
Cr(VI) 84
Cu/Zn superoxide dismutase 47
Cyclooxygenase 2 84
Cyclophosphamide (CP/CY) 82, 83, 93-96
Cyclosporine 93, 95
CYP2E1 57, 74

D

D195V 40
Dehydroascorbic acid (DHA) 47
DHPLC analysis 14
Diepoxybutane (DEB) 2, 5, 6, 14, 36, 37, 44, 67, 74, 82, 83, 85, 103
DNA 1, 2, 5-7, 9, 14, 18, 19, 21, 28, 31, 32, 36, 37, 42, 43, 46, 48, 55-58, 61-64, 67, 70, 71, 74-76, 78, 82-87, 93, 96, 97, 103, 104, 106, 108, 109, 111
DNA crosslinking agent 1, 2, 5-7, 9, 36, 46, 67, 83, 93, 97, 103
DNA damaging agents 57, 70, 96, 97
DNA double strand break (DSB) 1, 2, 18, 46
DNA excision repair 1
DNA interstrand crosslinks 2, 46, 70, 111
DNA repair 2, 18, 19, 21, 31, 32, 36, 37, 55, 58, 64, 76, 78, 82, 84, 86, 87, 96, 103
DNA repair/cell cycle checkpoint 55
DNA-dependent ATPase 75
Drosophila 61
dsRNA 17, 36, 46

E

E3 ubiquitin ligase activity 62
E417L 40
Electron paramagnetic resonance (EPR) 84
Endochondral ossification 40
Endocrine abnormalities 82, 85
Epidermal growth factor (EGF) 76
ERCC1 21, 78, 112
Ethnic background 30
European Blood and Marrow Transplantation (EBMT) Group 93, 94
European Fanconi Anemia Registry (EUFAR) 93
Exon 3 15, 108
Exon 3 (176-307del) 108
Exon 4 16, 32, 39, 40, 108
Exon 7 108, 109
Exon 8 15, 43, 109, 110
Exon 8 (1059-1076del) 109
Exon 15
Exon 22 106

Index

F

FA knockout mice 15
FA patients in Asian countries 103
FA-A patient 7, 8, 28-31, 54, 107-109
FA-C 7, 8, 17, 30, 36, 37, 39, 40, 42-49, 54, 67, 74, 75, 85, 103, 111
FA-C lymphoblastoid cell line (FA-C LCL) 36, 37, 40, 42, 43, 45-48
FA-G 7, 8, 17, 30, 54, 56, 57, 69, 109, 111, 112
FA20P 104, 105
FA33P 104
FAAP95 2
FANCA 2, 6, 8, 10, 13-17, 19-21, 28-33, 42, 54-57, 61-64, 67-71, 74-78, 82, 84, 97, 103-108, 111, 112
FANCA exon 43 10
FANCA kinase 14
FANCA locus 105, 106
Fanca murine models 32
FANCA null mutation 30
FANCA phosphorylation 31, 32, 55, 77
FANCA-BRG1-BRCA1 75
FANCB 2, 13-15, 20-22, 31, 55, 56, 58, 71, 111
FANCC 2, 6-8, 10, 13-21, 29-31, 33, 36-49, 54-57, 61-63, 67-70, 71, 74, 75, 82, 84, 85, 97, 98, 103, 110, 111
FANCC cDNA 40, 43, 44, 46, 111
FANCC exon 14 7
Fancc-/- mice 44-48
Fancc+/- 44, 45
Fancc+/+ 44, 46
*FANCC*322delG mutation 8
FANCD1 1, 2, 4, 7, 9, 10, 13, 14, 16, 18, 21, 55-58, 61, 63, 64, 68, 69, 103, 111
FANCD2 1, 2, 6, 7, 9, 10, 13-16, 18-22, 28, 33, 36, 41, 42, 46, 55-58, 61-64, 67-71, 75, 76, 78, 87, 103, 111
FANCD2 ubiquitination 14, 20, 64
FANCE 2, 6, 13, 14, 16, 19, 21, 31, 42, 48, 55-57, 62, 63, 67-70, 103, 111
FANCF 2, 6, 13, 14, 19, 20, 31, 42, 55-57, 62, 63, 67-69, 71, 98, 103, 111
FANCF ORF 57
FANCG 2, 3, 6, 13, 14, 16-21, 31, 33, 42, 55-57, 61-64, 67-71, 74, 75, 82, 84, 85, 103, 108-112

FANCG/CYP2E1 57
FANCG/XRCC9 56
FANCI 2, 14, 20, 55, 103
FANCJ 2, 7, 9, 14, 20, 55, 103
FANCL 2, 6, 13-15, 20, 22, 28, 42, 55, 61-63, 69-71, 103
FANCL/PHF9 70, 71
FANCM 2, 103
Fanconi anemia (FA) 1-10, 13-22, 28-33, 36-40, 42-49, 52-58, 61-65, 67-71, 74-76, 78, 79, 82-88, 92-98, 103-105, 107-109, 111, 112
Fanconi anemia zinc finger (FAZF) 16, 42, 74, 75
Fas ligand 17
Fas ligation 36, 47, 48
Fas receptor (CD95) 44, 45
Fas-mediated cell death 45
Fas-priming by IFN 47
Flavin mononucleotide (FMN) 47
Fludarabine 95, 96, 98
Frameshift 7, 15, 28, 39, 40, 104, 105, 110
Frameshift mutation 7, 28, 40, 104, 105
Free radical 43, 47, 55, 57, 86
Fungal infections 95

G

g. 1066C>T 110
G1/S 41
G2 phase of the cell cycle 36
G2/M 41-43, 75, 97
Gamma-irradiation 32, 41, 47
Gene therapy 96-98
Genotype-phenotype data 30, 32
Glucose intolerance 86
Glutathione (GSH) 47, 74, 83, 84, 86
Glutathione S-transferase 47, 74, 83, 84
Glutathione S-transferase (GSTP1) P1-1 16-18, 47-49, 74
Graft versus host disease (GVHD) 93-96
Granulocyte-colony stimulating factor (G-CSF) 92, 93, 97
Grd19p 76
GRP94 15, 16, 41, 75

H

3-hybrid 56, 69
8-hydroxy deoxy guanosine (8-OHdG) 57, 84, 85
70kDa heat shock protein (HSP70) 16, 17, 46, 48, 49, 84
Haplotype analysis 18, 104
Heat shock responses 20
Hematological correction 96
Hematopoiesis 3, 15-18, 22, 28-30, 32, 36, 40-45, 47, 48, 55, 75, 86, 92-94, 96-98
Hematopoietic cells 16-18, 22, 41, 45, 47, 94, 96-98
Hematopoietic stem cell (HPC) 29, 30, 36, 41, 43-45, 48, 49, 92-94, 96-98
Hematopoietic growth factor 92, 93
Heme oxygenase 83
Hepatic tumors 92
Hexavalent chromium compounds 82
HIV-1 97
HIV-2 97
HLA-matched sibling 92, 93, 96
HMRE11 2, 5
Homologous recombination (HR) 2, 19, 21, 32, 63, 68, 70, 71, 79, 112
Homologous recombination repair 2, 19, 21, 68, 79
Homozygous null (Fancc-/-) mice 43
HSC536 36, 39, 45, 46
HSC536 cell line 39, 46
HSC536 FA-C cell line 39
Human immunodeficiency virus (HIV) 96, 97
Hydrogen peroxide (H_2O_2) 18, 41, 47, 48, 57, 85
Hydroxyl radicals 83
Hygromycin 20
Hyperglycaemia 85
Hyperinsulinaemia 86
Hypogonadism 17
Hypomorphs 63
Hypothyroidism 86
Hypoxic 47

I

I312V 40
ICL 41, 42, 46, 48, 111, 112
IFN receptor-α 45
IκB kinase 15, 76
IKK 15, 76-79
IKK complex 76, 77, 79
IKK signalsome 76, 78
IKK2 15, 75, 76
IL-3 45, 98
Immunodeficiency 5, 6, 96, 98
Immunosuppressive agent 95, 96
Insertional mutagenesis 98
Interferon gamma (IFN-γ) 17, 41, 44-49, 75, 85, 97
International Bone Marrow Transplant Registry (IBMTR) 93
International Fanconi Anemia Registry (IFAR) 3, 111
Intragenic deletions 14
Intron 4 7, 39, 40
Intronless 19
Ionizing radiation (IR) 1, 2, 6, 7, 9, 10, 19, 47, 62, 63, 70, 75
IVS3+1G>C 20, 108, 109, 111, 112
IVS4 + 4 A>T 39, 40
IVS8-2A>G 110
IVS13-1G>C 109
IVS13-2A>G 108, 109
IVS27-1G>A 104, 106
IVS27-2A>T 104, 106
IVS41-2A>G 104, 106

J

Jak kinase 17
Japanese FA 10, 103, 104, 107, 109, 111, 112
JNK 47, 48

L

L190F 40
LCL 36, 37, 40, 46
Lentivirus 96, 97
Lentivirus HIV-1 97
Lentivirus HIV-2 97
Leukemia 1, 3, 4, 9, 10, 13, 32, 33, 54, 62, 75, 85, 86, 95, 96, 98

Lipid peroxidation 83, 84
Lipoxygenase 86
LMO2 gene locus 98
Lymphoblasts 37, 45, 46, 54, 56, 57, 67, 84
Lymphopaenia 5
Lymphoproliferative malignancies 96

M

8-methoxypsoralen 82, 84
Macrophage inflammatory protein-1α (MIP-1α) 17, 44, 97
MAPKKK 48
Mass spectroscopy 62
Medulloblastoma 4, 8, 9
MEFs 45, 46, 48
Melatonin 84
Microcell fusions 61
Microdeletions 14, 29
Microinsertions 14
Microophthalmia 32
Mismatch repair 64
Missense mutation 7, 9, 39, 104, 105
Mitomycin C (MMC) 2, 5, 6, 8, 14, 18-20, 22, 32, 36, 37, 39-47, 49, 54-57, 62, 63, 67, 69, 70, 74, 82, 83, 85, 93, 97, 98, 103, 111
Mitosis 21, 41, 42, 75
Modulatory role 68
Monoubiquitination 2, 6, 7, 9, 13, 15, 21, 28, 36, 41, 42, 46, 57, 61-64, 87
Mosaicism 7, 18, 29, 97
Mouse cells 9
MRE11 21, 46, 55, 68, 112
Multigenic disorder 13
Murine leukemia virus (MLV) 96
Mutation 1-3, 5-10, 13-22, 28-30, 32, 33, 39-42, 45, 46, 49, 54-56, 61-64, 67-71, 93, 103-112
Mutation Q13X 39
Mutation W22X 39
Mvp1p 76
Myelodysplasia 13, 93
Myelodysplastic syndrome (MDS) 3, 4, 7, 8, 40
Myelogenous leukemia 32, 85

N

N-acetylcysteine 83, 84
NADPH 16, 47, 74, 84
NADPH cytochrome P450 reductase 74, 84
Nbs1 protein 5, 7
Nephroblastoma 4
Neutrophil 92, 93
NF-κB 57, 76, 77, 79
Nijmegen breakage syndrome (NBS) 1, 2, 5-7, 21, 46, 47, 55, 62, 68, 112
Nitric oxide (NO) 47, 48
Nitrogen mustard 43
Nonerythroid α spectrin 112
NonFanconi aplastic anemia 96
Nonpathogenic polymorphic variants 107
NSP2 57
Nuclear translocation 16, 21
Null mutations 2, 18, 30, 54, 68

O

Oligodeoxynucleotide 43
Oxidative stress 14, 17, 18, 20, 47, 74, 82-87
Oxygen 47, 74, 82, 83, 85
Oxymethalone 4, 92

P

26S proteasome 41
P211R 40
p38 signalling cascades 48
P450 47, 57, 74, 84, 86
P450 2E1 57, 74, 84
p53 37, 39, 43-45, 48, 75, 87
Pancytopenia 3, 54, 86
Patient AP78M 106
Patient FA20P 104
PHD finger protein-9 (PHF9) 14, 20, 69, 70, 71
PHD-type E3 ubiquitin ligase 70
Phosphatidylinositol-3 kinase 31, 32
Phosphatidylinositol-3,4,5-trisphosphate 77
Phosphoinositide (PI) 76, 77
Phosphoinositide 3-kinase (PI-3K) 77
Phosphoinositide-dependent kinase-1 (PDK-1) 77
Phosphoprotein 39, 56
Phosphorylation 9, 14, 15, 31, 32, 39, 46, 47, 55, 63, 70, 75, 77-79
PKC phosphorylation 39

PKR 16-18, 20, 46, 48, 49
   see also RNA-dependent protein kinase
Placental blood program 94
Plasmid DNA 46
Polymorphic site 104-107, 109
Polymorphism 28-30, 38, 40, 55, 107, 109, 111
Post-translational modification 14, 28, 70
Preintegration complex 96
Pro-oxidant state 82-86
Promyelocytic leukemia zinc finger (PLZF) 42, 75
Prostaglandin H synthase 86
Protein ROM 19, 57
Psoralen + UVA 42, 43
PUVA 82, 84
PX 76
Pyrimidine dimers 1

Q

Q465R 40

R

RAD50 46, 55, 68, 112
Rad51 16, 18, 19, 21, 22, 47, 56, 58, 62, 63, 69, 70
Rad54 21
Radiation therapy 93, 96, 97
Reactive oxygen species (ROS) 47, 74, 76, 83, 84, 86
RecQ helicase 70
RED 47, 49, 74
Redox cycling 47, 74, 82
Redox regulation 18, 76
Redox state 36, 47, 49, 84, 87
Redox-related toxicity 82
Restriction site of Cac8I 107
Retroviral 44, 45, 96-98
Retroviral vector 96-98
Retrovirus 6, 44, 97
Rev3 21
RFLP analysis 104, 107, 108
RMN assembly 46
RNA splicing mutation 105
RNA-dependent protein kinase 20, 46
   see also PKR
ROM 19, 57
RPA 14/32/70 64
RPA1 19
Rutin 83

S

S-phase 2, 9, 16, 19, 21, 41-43, 46, 48, 62, 70
S-phase checkpoint 9, 46
S26F 40
SCID 98
SCID mouse xenotransplant 98
Seckel syndrome 5
Semiquinone radicals 83
Serine 222 9, 63
Serine kinase 14, 71
Serine phosphorylation of FANCA 31
Serine-threonine kinase 48
Signal-regulating kinase 1 48
Skin pigmentation 3-6, 82, 85, 86
Snm1 21
SNX1 76
SNX5 16, 75-78
Sod1 47
Somatic mosaicism 29, 97
Splicing mutation 14, 105, 109, 110
Squamous cell carcinoma 4, 95
STAT 17, 18, 46
STAT molecules 17
STAT1 phosphorylation 46, 75
STAT1 signaling 45
Stem cell transplantation 62, 92, 93
Stoichiometry of FA proteins 31
Superoxide dismutase (SOD) 47, 83
SWI/SNF 15, 75, 76, 78, 79

T

T cell leukaemia 4, 9, 10
T-cell 17, 94, 95, 98
TATA box 37
Testosterone 92
TGF-β 41
Thalidomide 86
Thioredoxin (Trx) 83, 85, 86
Thoracoabdominal 93, 94
Thrombocytopenia 95
Thrombocytosis 5
Tip60 21
TNF receptor 45
Transgene 96-98
Tumor necrosis factor alpha (TNFα) 17, 44-46, 49, 57, 76, 77, 85, 97
Tyk2 17
Type II diabetes mellitus 82

U

Ubiquitin ligase 2, 15, 20, 28, 61, 62, 70
Ultraviolet (UV) light 1, 82

V

V449M 40
V60I 40
Viral vectors 96, 97
Vitamin C 83
Vps5p 76

W

Wilms tumour 4, 9

X

X-linked FA 15
Xeroderma pigmentosum (XP) 1, 2
Xp22.31 14, 15, 58
XPF 21, 70, 78
XRCC2 21
XRCC3 21
XRCC9 2, 20, 56

Y

Yeast 2-hybrid 56, 57, 69
Yeast 3-hybrid 56